Dr James Witchalls MB, BS, D Obst RCOG

The original edition of this book was written by James Witchalls who graduated from St Bartholomew's Hospital, in the City of London, in 1967. Since that time he has worked in hospital practice for three years including 18 months in the Albert Schweitzer Hospital in Gabon, West Africa, where he was mainly concerned with children. He has also worked for 10 years in General Practice in England where his main interest has been in maternity and child health. He has lectured extensively on First Aid and has participated in many conferences concerned with the health of children.

Aquatic Safety Group

This new edition has been completely revised and updated by the Aquatic Safety Group in conjunction with the NSW Ambulance Training Board. The Aquatic Safety Group is an organisation dealing with safety in the aquatic environment. It has broad experience in water safety and Emergency Water First Aid and is committed to educating the community on aquatic safety.

It offers courses in Paediatric First Aid which can be held at schools or in the home if there are more than six participants. The course is CPR certified.

Contents

Introduction

Childhood accidents are more common today than ever before and a greater proportion of children die as a result of accidents than from any other single cause. This is partly because deaths from other causes have been drastically reduced during the past 50 years as medical science has made it possible for us to protect our children from a range of previously fatal diseases, such as diphtheria, whooping cough and pneumonia. Parallel with this desirable development, however, has been a corresponding increase in the exposure of children to mechanical and electrical appliances, such as motor cars, bicycles, electric kettles and fires, and household products which can be poisonous to children if consumed, such as disinfectants, cleaning agents and petroleum products. There has never been a greater need, therefore, for vigilance and preparedness to meet the emergency.

As a parent and doctor, with a special interest in the health and welfare of children, I find it all too common today that young parents are not sufficiently aware of the increasing sources of accidents and quite unprepared to take the necessary First Aid steps to deal with accidents until medical help is available. After all, the parent carrying out efficient First Aid is as likely to reduce injury and save the life of a child as the most skilful medical attention. Although prevention must remain our best defence against childhood injuries, nothing can, nor should, stop children from reaching out to explore their environment. Therefore accidents will happen at times, even in the safest situations.

This book, then, is designed to act as a practical guide to parents, baby-sitters, teachers and others dealing with children who at some time, usually unexpectedly, will be faced with a child who has had an accident. However, please note that this is a guide only and medical help should always be sought as soon as possible.

The book will be most helpful to you if you familiarise yourself with the first section, Prepare Yourself, as soon as possible. **Do not wait for an accident to happen.** Always keep details of your children's medical history and a list of emergency telephone numbers and addresses – and keep them up-to-date. Use the section on the First Aid Kit as a guide to preparing your own – and keep it well stocked and easily accessible.

Mitchell

SECTION 1

Prepare yourself

Throughout this book symbols are used to indicate actions which must often be carried out in addition to basic first aid treatment. These may appear at the beginning of the sequence of actions, or at the end, depending upon the seriousness of the child's condition. They may also be used in conjunction. For example, where you are instructed to watch the child's breathing and give mouth-to-mouth resuscitation the symbols for checking breathing *and* emergency resuscitation or artificial ventilation will both appear.

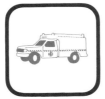
Remove to hospital

Check the breathing

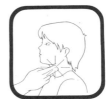
Check the pulse

Apply heart compression

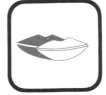
Apply artificial ventilation

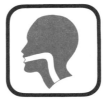
Clear the airway

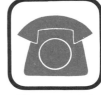
Summon medical aid

Emergency action

First Aid consists of certain approved methods of treating a sick or injured child until he or she is placed, if necessary, in the care of a doctor or removed to hospital.

When faced with such an emergency act in the following sequence:

First Aid has three principle aims:

- To sustain life
- To prevent the condition from worsening
- To promote recovery

1 ASSESSMENT

Be calm and take charge of the situation, acting confidently and reassuring the child. Make sure that there is no further danger to the child, yourself, or any others who may be present. **Check for consciousness, breathing, pulse and bleeding.**

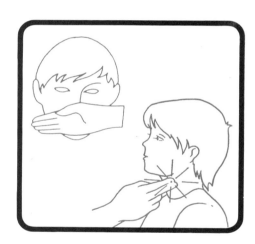

2 DIAGNOSIS

Find out what has happened — ask the child, if conscious, or a witness. In the event of illness, try to find out if the child has a history of illness. Examine for injury and record the level of consciousness, if necessary.

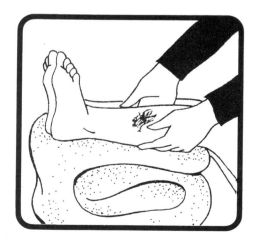

Emergency action

3 TREATMENT

Prevent the condition from becoming worse – cover wounds, immobilise fractures, place child in the correct and comfortable position. Promote recovery by reassuring, relieving pain, handling gently and carefully, protecting from cold.

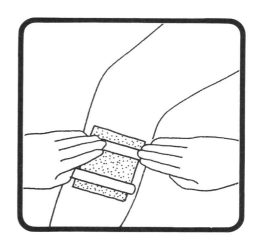

4 DISPOSAL

Ensure that the child is removed with minimum delay to home, suitable shelter or hospital. If necessary send a tactful message to the child's home stating the nature of accident or illness and where child has been removed to. Remove by ambulance unless the injury is a minor one.

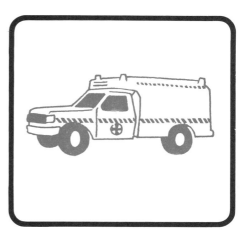

5 DO NOT

- Attempt too much
- Allow people to crowd around
- Remove the casualty's clothing unnecessarily
- Give anything by mouth to a child who is unconscious, has a suspected internal injury or may need an anaesthetic

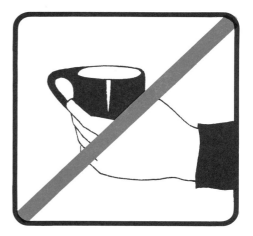

Resuscitation

IMPORTANT
The first and most vital aim of resuscitation is artificial ventilation (artificial breathing) which ensures that adequate air is getting to the lungs. Regular breathing must be established, or artificial ventilation continued, to ensure that oxygen-containing blood reaches all parts of the body, especially the brain.

Make sure breathing has stopped: Look and feel for movement of the lower chest and upper abdomen. Then, listen and feel for the escape of air from nose and mouth.

1 The unconscious victim's airway should be cleared quickly before assessment of breathing and circulation. With the victim lying on his side, the rescuer should use his fingers to clear the mouth of any visible objects: eg plastic, blood, vomit, teeth or a foreign object. Nostrils should also be cleared in infants.

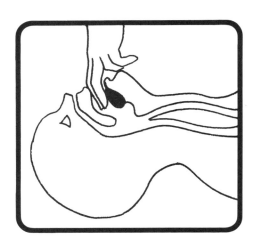

2 Lay the child flat on back on a firm surface; eg floor or table. Remove all pillows.

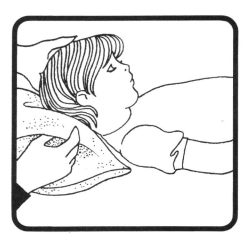

10

Resuscitation

3 INFANTS 0 - 1 YEAR

The head should be kept horizontal and your open mouth placed firmly over the infant's mouth and nose so there is no air gap around the edges of your mouth.

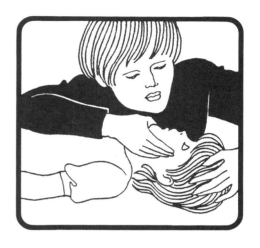

4

Give gentle puffs of air from your cheeks. Use just enough pressure to cause the infant's chest to rise. Remove mouth and watch chest fall. Continue at a rate of approximately one inflation every 3 seconds. Watch for spontaneous breathing. Repeat until breathing recommences.

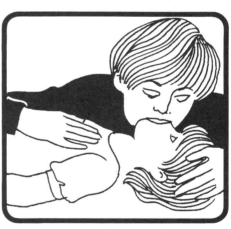

5 OLDER CHILDREN

Carry out the above procedure but place your open mouth over the child's mouth only. With one hand firmly pinch the child's nose to prevent air escaping through his nose. Take 3 seconds over each breath.

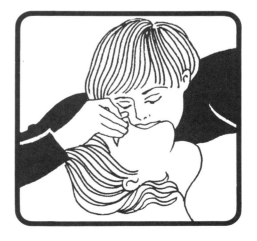

Resuscitation

IMPORTANT

If two first aiders are present there should be no pause compressions and the inflation should be interposed between the last compression of the cycle and the first of the next. DO NOT change the sequence or overlap your action.

Check for pulse (see page 14): if pulse is present but casualty is not breathing, continue to give artificial respiration until natural breathing recommences

1 After detecting the absence of the pulse, it is important to expose the chest and find the correct chest position for C.P.R. (cardiopulmonary resuscitation).

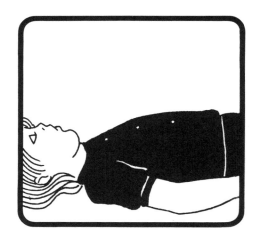

2 ## INFANTS

The rescuer should identify the lower end of the sternum and apply compression above this point. The fingers or hand should not extend beyond the end of the sternum.

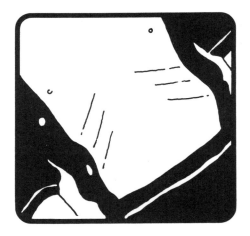

Resuscitation

3 Make short firm compressions down toward the backbone using two fingers only, compressing the sternum approximately 2 cm. The rate of inflation to compressions will be:

One rescuer — two inflations to fifteen compressions in 10 seconds, providing six cycles per minute.

Two rescuers — one inflation to five compressions in 3 seconds, providing twenty cycles per minute.

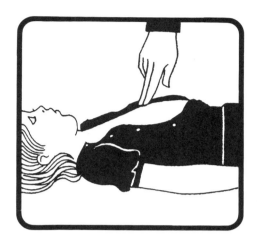

4 Check pulse initially after 1 minute and from then on every 2 minutes. Continue sequence until medical help arrives or the natural function of the lungs and heart returns.

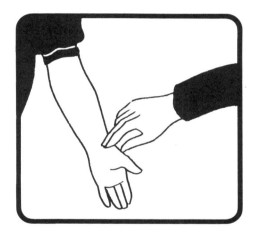

5 **OLDER CHILDREN**

Use the heel of one hand for the compressions otherwise the technique is the same as described for infants.

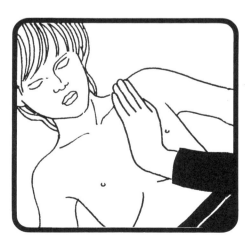

The pulse

IMPORTANT

The heart beats about 90 to 110 times each minute in a young child and about 80 to 100 times each minute in an older child. Each heartbeat forces blood around the arteries of the body and can be felt as a pressure wave over several points of the body.

There is no need to take the pulse for a whole minute. It should be sufficient to take it for 10 seconds and multiply the result by 6

1 The neck is the easiest place to feel the pulse. Place your index or middle finger on the side of the neck next to the windpipe and gently press towards the rear. Use tips of fingers NOT thumb.

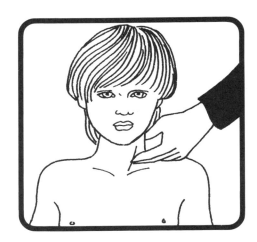

2 Gently press the tips of your index and middle fingers over the under side of the wrist at the base of the thumb

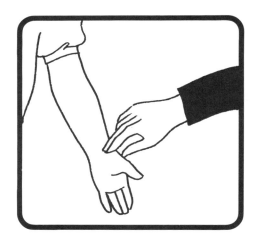

The pulse

3 ARM: Place index and middle finger on inside of elbow, towards thumb side of arm.

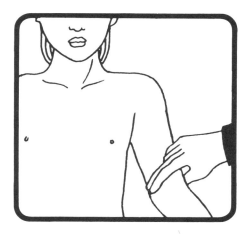

4 GROIN: Gently press your index and middle fingers over the middle of the groin fold.

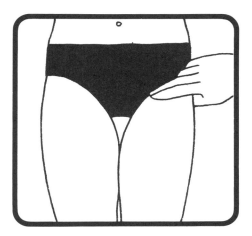

Unconsciousness

The first stage of unconsciousness is *drowsiness*, from which the child may be easily roused; the next stage is *stupor*, from which the child may be roused only with difficulty; the most serious and advanced stage is *coma*, from which the child cannot be roused at all. Unless the child is fully alert, treat as if unconscious.

The first aim, in dealing with any unconscious child, is to ensure an open airway and summon immediate medical aid

1 Check airway, breathing and pulse.

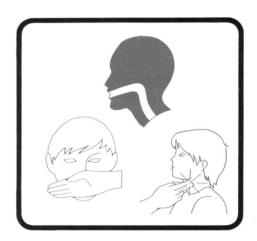

2 Loosen clothing around the neck, chest and waist and ensure that plenty of fresh air is available.

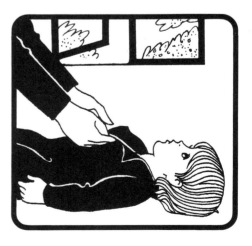

Unconsciousness

3 Lay child in the position shown here – the Recovery Position – preferably with the lower part of the body slightly raised above the head. This will ensure that vomit or saliva does not flow into the lungs. Do not provide pillows and keep the head flexed slightly backwards.

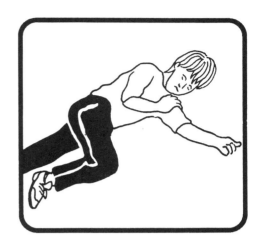

4 Cover with a blanket to maintain body temperature but do not over heat. Stay with the child until medical help arrives. Never leave an unconscious child unattended.

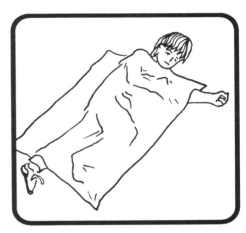

5 If consciousness returns, speak reassuringly to the child, and prevent him from hurting himself. If thirsty, moisten lips, DO NOT attempt to give a drink to an unconscious child.

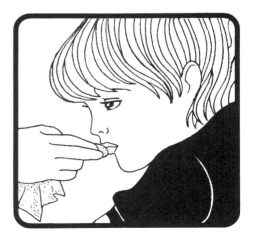

Temperature

IMPORTANT

The normal body temperature is 37.5°C (98.4°F), but it may vary by ½°C (1°F) without indicating any abnormality. Those slight variations may occur, for example, in the early morning (lower) or in very hot weather, after severe exertion or after hot meals (higher). Feeling the skin gives only a general guide to body temperature.

If the body temperature is below 36°C (96.8°F) or above 39.5°C (103°F), seek medical advice

When warmed, the mercury in the bulb of the thermometer expands and pushes up through the narrow hollow centre of the thermometer. It shrinks on cooling. Rotate the thermometer slowly between your fingers until you see the tip of the column of mercury against the scale on the side. Electronic thermometers are safer, quicker, more accurate and easier to read. They are readily available at chemists.

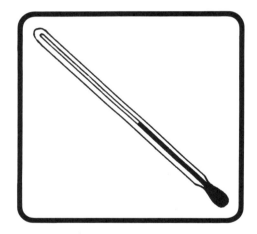

UNDER THE ARM: Place the bulb of the thermometer high under the armpit and support it by pressing the child's arm against its chest. Read after about 2 minutes. *This method usually shows a temperature ½°C (1°F) lower than normal.*

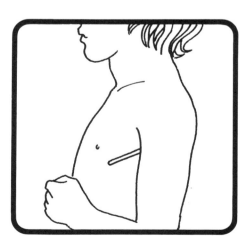

Abnormally low temperatures are frequently brought about by shock, severe bleeding or exposure

Temperature

IN THE GROIN: Place the bulb of the thermometer in the skin fold of the groin and gently hold the legs of the child together. Read after 2 minutes. *This method usually shows a temperature ½°C (1°F) lower than normal.*

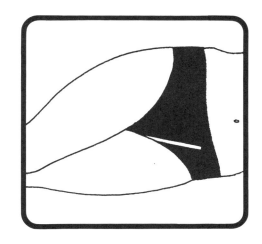

IN THE MOUTH: (Suitable in children over 5 years old.) Place the bulb of the thermometer under one side of the tongue on the floor of the mouth. Support the thermometer between gently closed lips. Read after 2 minutes.

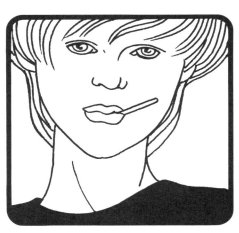

IN THE RECTUM: (At any age but especially in babies and infants.) Use a plastic rectal thermometer. Gently slip the bulb of the thermometer through the anus into the rectum (about 25mm) and support it there for 1 minute. *This will result in a temperature reading ½°C (1°F) higher than normal.*

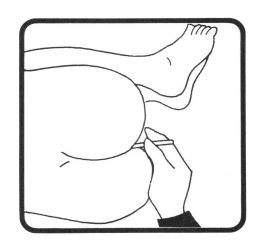

Abnormally high temperatures occur during 'teething' and a variety of general body infections

First aid kit

The kit shown here is recommended for all households. Other items, not illustrated, may be added for special purposes, but for basic First Aid requirements this kit should be adequate. Keep it well stocked and replace the disposable items as they are used. Keep a separate kit in your car or boat and for hiking and camping.

BASIC KIT

1 Pocket resuscitation mask — this enables air to go one way only and also prevents you from inhaling blood or vomit from the patient. Keep a mask at home and in the car.
2 Adhesive strip plasters — assorted sizes.
3 Adhesive tape — 12mm or 25mm wide.
4 Calamine lotion.
5 Cotton tipped swabs.
6 Children's aspirin/paracetamol — according to doctor's advice — but not for infants under 1 year old.
7 Antiseptic solution.
8 Oil of cloves — for minor toothache.
9 Rubbing alcohol or Cologne.
10 Triangular bandages — for tying splints.
11 Safety pins.
12 Sharp needles — to remove splinters: sterilise first.
13 Sharp scissors with rounded ends.
14 Sterile eye pads.
15 Sterile gauze bandages — 25mm and 50mm.
16 Sterile gauze pads — 50mm and 100mm square.
17 Thermometer.
18 Tongue depressors — wooden.
19 Tweezers.

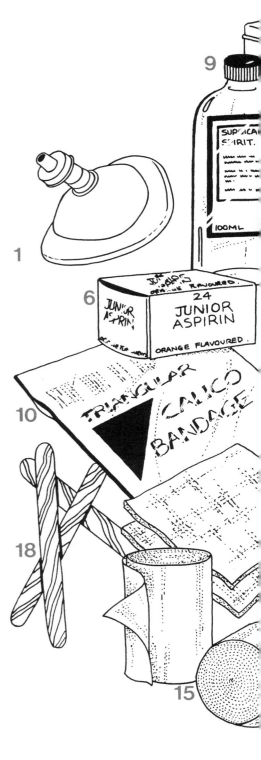

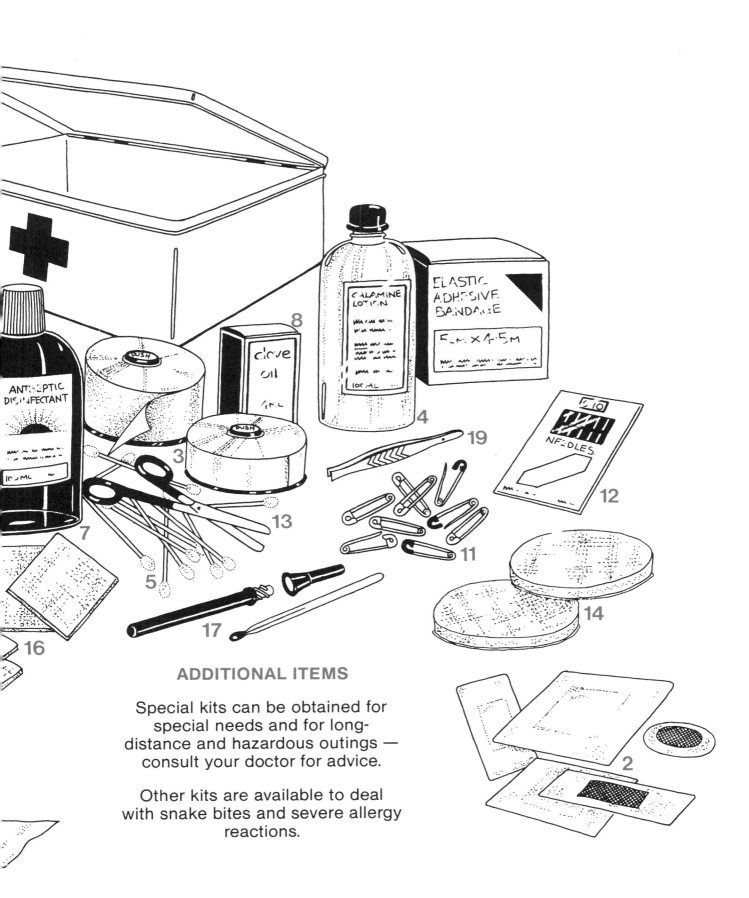

ADDITIONAL ITEMS

Special kits can be obtained for special needs and for long-distance and hazardous outings — consult your doctor for advice.

Other kits are available to deal with snake bites and severe allergy reactions.

Bandages

Bandages may be made from flannel, calico, elastic net or special paper. They can also be improvised from any of these materials or from socks, stockings, ties, belts, scarves etc.

Bandages are used chiefly to control bleeding by maintaining direct pressure over a dressing and to retain dressings and splints in position. They may also be used to prevent and reduce swellings, to give support to a limb or joint, to restrict movement and assist in lifting or carrying casualties. *Never use bandages for padding when other materials are to hand.*

APPLICATION: Bandages must be applied firmly enough to control bleeding and to prevent dressings and splints from slipping. If they are too tight, circulation will be impeded and the underlying part injured. If the toes or fingers become white or blueish, or become numb, loosen the bandage a little.

TYING BANDAGES: All bandages of this type should be tied with a reef knot, which does not slip, is flat and is easy to untie. The knot should be placed away from the injured part and should not cause discomfort. For their various uses see page 84, Fractures.

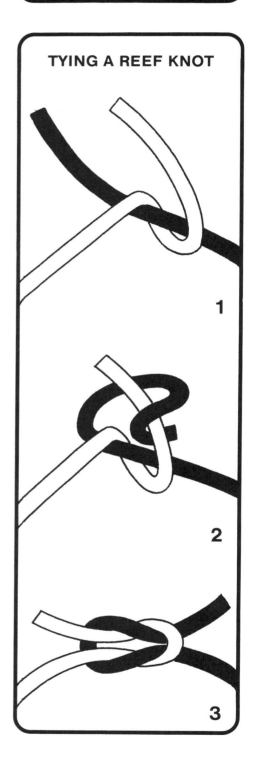

TYING A REEF KNOT

1

2

3

Bandages

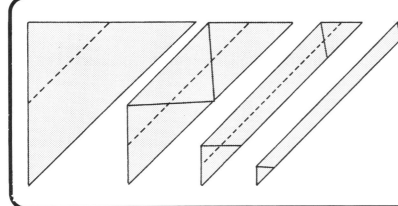

Triangular bandages can be made from squares of linen or calico – between 50cm and 1m square – cut diagonally into two pieces. They can be used as slings or folded to make either broad or narrow bandages.

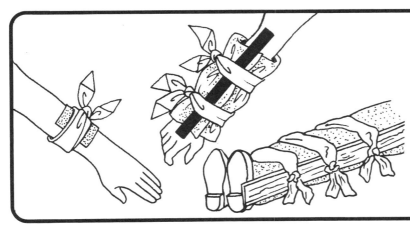

Narrow bandages are not only useful for binding wounds and holding dressings in position, they are ideal for tying around splints and protective padding.

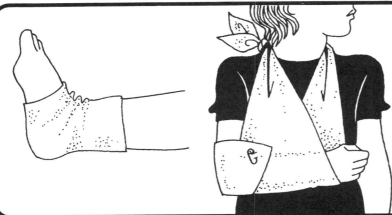

Elasticated bandages can be used to support injured joints – sprained ankles or wrists, for example. Slings can be bought ready-made or they can be adapted from triangular bandages.

Dressings

A dressing should be germ free (sterile), if possible, and able to act as a filter – restricting entry of germs but allowing air to reach the wound. It must also be very porous in order to absorb blood and sweat. If sweat cannot evaporate through it, an infection can set in. It should also be of a non-adherent material so that it will not damage the repairing wound.

A dressing is a protective covering applied to a wound to control bleeding, prevent infection, absorb blood and discharge and prevent further damage

Adhesive dressings : These are often called 'plasters'; eg band aids and consist of a pad of absorbent gauze or cellulose with an adhesive backing which, if perforated, allows sweat to evaporate. The surrounding skin should be dry before application. When a dressing has no sticking power of its own it must be held in place by a bandage.

Prepared sterile dressings consist of layers of gauze covered by a pad of cotton wool and come with a roller bandage to tie them in position.

Plain gauze dressings come in a variety of sizes. They tend to stick to wounds but this can assist in clotting.

Vaseline gauze dressings are sold in squares in sealed packs. They are available in a number of different sizes and they do not stick to wounds.

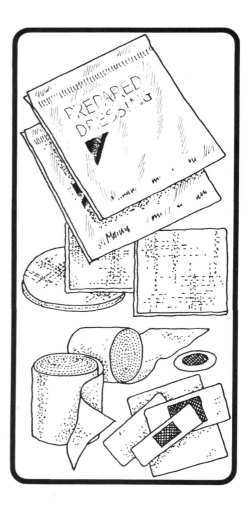

Dressings

IMPROVISED DRESSINGS

These are important because accidents tend to happen when and where ideal equipment is not available. Dressings may be improvised from clean hankies, freshly laundered towels or linen or any other clean absorbent material. Keep them in position with whatever material is to hand.

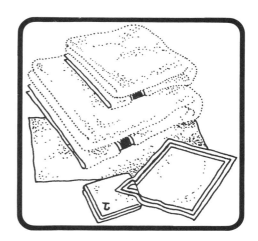

HANDLING DRESSINGS

Wash your hands before handling dressings and bandages, and avoid touching wounds with fingers. Dressings should be covered with adequate padding, extending well beyond the wound and held in place with a bandage.

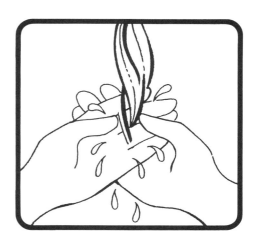

CREAM AND OINTMENTS

In general, minor wounds are best cleaned with soap and water — creams and ointments should be unnecessary. Infected wounds need an antiseptic solution which can be obtained from your chemist. Antibiotic medication can only be obtained from your doctor.

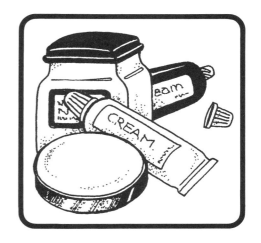

Seek medical advice if you are in doubt about the use of any application

25

Aids to survival

HEAT

Do not undergo strenuous exertion during the hottest period of the day. Drink more water than usual and take salt tablets if necessary. A rest after lunch, in the shade, should be encouraged.

Acclimatise gradually before sudden exposure to heat, especially moist heat

Wear loose cotton clothing over the whole of the trunk and a lightweight hat with a broad brim of at least 10 cm or legionnaires-style cap. Sunscreen of 15+ SPF and/or sunblock should also be used. Open shoes or sandals will also be beneficial.

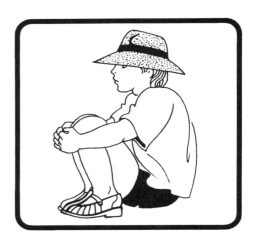

COLD

If possible, acclimatise gradually to conditions of extreme cold. Wear several layers of light woollen or cotton over-garments and soft woollen underclothing. Several light layers are better than one thick, heavy garment.

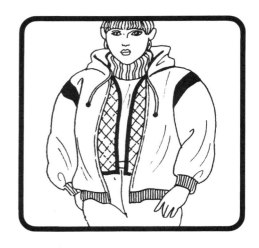

26

Aids to survival

Cover the extremities of the body, hands head and ears and wear comfortable, waterproof leather shoes or boots.

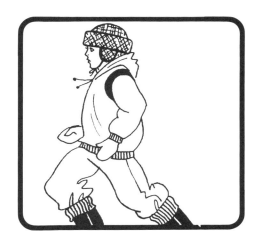

Do not sit or stand around in cold conditions and have plenty of warm drinks and high calorie foods.

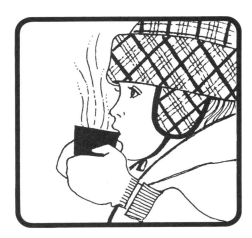

Remove wet clothing as soon as possible if shelter is available. On hikes or walks, carry a large plastic bag and/or a space blanket large enough to accommodate a child suffering from exposure.

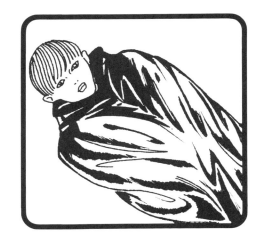

Children should be encouraged to wear brightly coloured garments so that they may be easily seen

27

Aids to survival

Water in all forms attracts children, but any water of a greater depth than a few centimetres presents considerable dangers. If you always observe the following rules, however, your children should be able to enjoy water safely.

Teach your children to swim as soon as possible

- Avoid unsupervised exposure of young children to water any deeper than 5cm. Never leave a baby alone near water for a moment – a drowning accident can happen in seconds.
- If the telephone rings while bathing baby, wrap him in towel and carry with you to telephone. Similarly when answering the door bell.
- Never let infants or young children play around cesspools, puddles, ditches, wells or buckets of water.
- Keep swimming pools covered with hard cover during months when not in use.
- Forbid your young children to enter neighbours' swimming pools unless permission is given.
- Never let a toddler run loose near a pool.
- Know of the depth of a pool before letting your child enter the water.
- Encourage your child to use inflated tubes, rafts or armbands under supervision
- Never let your child go swimming alone.
- Never allow a child to get out of its depth unless well able to swim.
- Keep all children out of boats unless supervised.
- Supervise all fishing expeditions – never let a child go fishing alone.
- Young children should always wear a life-jacket if taken out on a boating or canoeing trip.

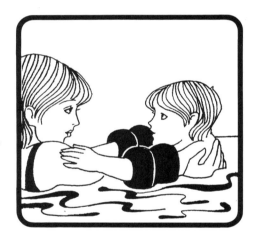

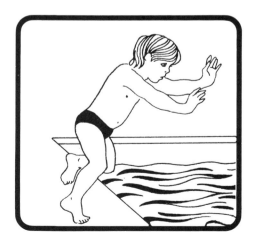

Rescue

1 Try to reach the child from land – using a hand, leg, clothing, pole, rope or anything that floats. If child is unconscious and not breathing, begin resuscitation at once. See page 10.

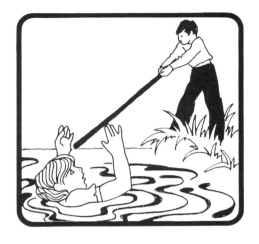

2 When rescuing older children from water, try to avoid being clutched by them as they struggle.

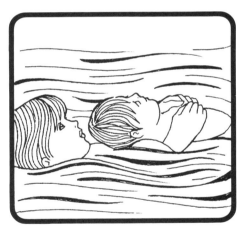

3 If you swim out to a child keep a close eye on the spot where you last saw the child. If possible take a life-buoy, or something that floats, with you for the child to hang on to.

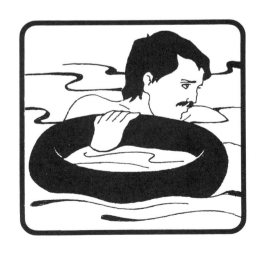

Never attempt a rescue in the water beyond your own swimming capability.

Childhood illnesses

ILLNESS	SYMPTOMS	INCUBATION	DURATION
● **Appendicitis** (Unusual under the age of 2 yrs)	Sudden onset of pain in centre of stomach, which moves after some hours to the lower right side; fever; vomiting; constipation; refusal of food.	None	Seek immediate medical attention
● **Chickenpox**	Fever accompanied by itchy pink or red spots on chest, back and stomach – sometimes spreading to scalp and face. These change to blisters and then crust.	10 to 21 days	7 to 10 days
● **Croup**	Laboured breathing accompanied by loud barking cough and hoarseness. Often comes on at night.	2 to 6 days	4 to 5 days
● **German Measles** (*Rubella*)	Painful swelling of glands behind the ears accompanied by low or high fever, chills and runny nose. Usually there is a fine red rash, which begins on the face and spreads over entire body.	14 to 21 days	3 to 6 days
● **Measles**	Early symptoms include low fever accompanied by slight hacking cough, fatigue, discomfort and eye irritation. Around the 4th day, fever and cough worsen and rash of faint pink spots appears on neck and cheeks then spreads to rest of body.	10 to 15 days	8 to 12 days
● **Mumps**	Swollen gland on one or both sides of the upper neck accompanied by headache and fever.	12 to 24 days	6 to 10 days
● **Pneumonia**	Coughing plus fever; rapid breathing; discomfort; chills and weakness; possible nausea and vomiting; sudden fever lasting several days.	2 to 14 days	About 7 days
● **Scarlet Fever**	Painful sore throat accompanied by fever; nausea and vomiting. Within 3 days a fine rash appears on neck, armpit and groin, then spreads over body.	1 to 5 days	6 to 8 days
● **Tonsillitis** (*Pharyngitis in babies*)	Painful sore throat; fever; tender swollen glands under sides of jaw; refusal to eat and drink; nausea and vomiting.	2 to 5 days	About 5 to 7 days
● **Whooping Cough** (*Pertussis*)	Dry persistent cough for 7 to 14 days becoming a whoop in older children; watery runny nose; child distressed and exhausted; vomiting.	7 to 10 days	Several weeks

30

INFECTIOUS FOR	TREATMENT	PRECAUTIONS
Not infectious	Seek immediate medical attention; give nothing to eat or drink.	
1 day before spots appear to about 6 days after	Consult your doctor. Rest is essential; calamine will relieve itching.	Keep all utensils separate.
2 days before symptoms appear to 5 days after	Consult your doctor. Use a vaporizer and keep child on a light, low fat diet.	
7 days before symptoms appear to 5 days after. Dangerous to pregnant women	If the child has fever, make sure he rests and supply plenty of juice.	Keep child's hands clean. Launder linen and clothes separately.
4 days before rash appears to 5 days after	Consult your doctor. If child's eyes are sensitive to light, keep the room dim. If fever occurs make sure he rests and give him plenty of juice.	Keep all utensils and dishes separate.
7 days before symptoms appear to 5 days after	Consult your doctor. Rest is essential. Apply cool compresses to the cheeks. Do not give citrus juices.	
Varies	Consult your doctor. Make sure the child rests and give him plenty of fluids.	Keep all utensils and dishes separate
1 day before symptoms appear to 6 days after	Consult your doctor. Make sure child rests and give plenty of fluids.	Check other family members for symptoms.
From day of onset until throat clears, about 7 days	Consult your doctor. Usually antibiotics given.	Keep eating and drinking utensils and toothbrush separate.
From 4 days before onset until 28 days after onset	Seek medical attention and follow advice.	Small frequent feeds to reduce chance of vomiting.

● After infection, immunity to re-infection usually lasts through childhood

31

Immunisation

These days all children can and should be protected against a number of serious infectious diseases. You are strongly advised to have all your children immunised against the following diseases at all times indicated. Consult your doctor, health visitor, Child Welfare Clinic or Baby Health Centre for advice.

This schedule is meant as a guide only — if in doubt seek medical advice

AGE	DISEASE	AGENT
2 months	Pertussis-Diptheria-Tetanus Poliomyelitis	Triple Antigen* Sabin Oral Vaccine
4 months	Pertussis-Diptheria-Tetanus Poliomyelitis	Triple Antigen* Sabin Oral Vaccine
6 months	Pertussis-Diptheria-Tetanus Poliomyelitis	Triple Antigen* Sabin Oral Vaccine
12 months	Measles	Measles virus vaccine, live attenuated (Schwarz strain)
18 months	Diptheria-Tetanus	Diptheria and Tetanus Toxoid Vaccine (CDT)
School entry	Diptheria-Tetanus Poliomyelitis	Diptheria and Tetanus Toxoid Vaccine (CDT) Sabin Oral Vaccine

*Pertussis (Whooping Cough) vaccine or Triple Antigen should not be used, but replaced by CDT for children with the following:
1 A previous history of neurological disease, including seizures, convulsions or cerebral irritation in the neonatal period.
2 A previous reaction to the vaccine other than minor local reactions and/or mild fever.
These children should be given CDT injections at 4 months, 6 months and 18 months of age.

- If there is a measles epidemic consult your doctor
- If you plan to travel abroad with your child consult your doctor well in advance
- If your child has a large skin wound, consult your doctor about the need for a Tetanus booster injection

32

SECTION 2
What to do

In this section you will find practical instruction on how to deal with a wide range of emergencies. Each important stage of treatment is accompanied by an explicit illustration or by a symbol referring to one of the life-saving methods explained in Section 1. Reading the book through *before* an emergency occurs is not only advisable, but necessary — you cannot deal with a serious burn, for example, with your First Aid manual propped up like a cookery book!

35

Asphyxia

SYMPTOMS OF ASPHYXIA

Breathing: Rate, depth and difficulty increase and later breathing becomes noisy with frothing at the mouth. Finally, breathing stops.

Congestion: The head and neck, face, lips and whites of eyes become red and eventually turn purple. Finger and toenail beds become purple.

Heartbeat: Becomes fast, then weak and finally stops.

Unconsciousness: Drowsiness is followed by stupor, then unrousable coma ending in death.

The commonest causes of asphyxia are spasms of the breathing tract, obstruction of the airway, suffocation and conditions which prevent oxygen use by the body. *Spasms* may be caused by food, water, smoke, irritant gases, asthma and some chest infections.

Obstruction of the airway may be caused by swallowed foreign bodies, food, teeth, blood, vomit, swellings and even the child's tongue falling back when unconscious. *Suffocation* may be caused by pillows and plastic bags and *oxygen use* may be impeded by car exhausts, gas supplies, chemical fumes and smoke.

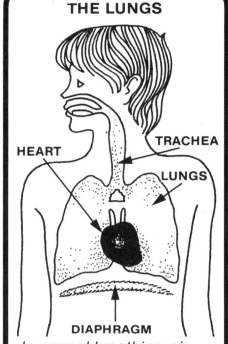

THE LUNGS

HEART — TRACHEA — LUNGS — DIAPHRAGM

In normal breathing, air passes through the windpipe into the lungs. The diaphragm, during inhaling, moves down and flattens out causing a partial vacuum in the lungs. Air is drawn in to equalise the pressure. During exhaling, the elastic tissue of the walls of the lungs enables them to deflate. Asphyxia occurs when an adequate supply of oxygen is not available to the body's blood supply. It may be due to a shortage of oxygen in the air breathed or to inadequate functioning of the heart and lungs.

Asphyxia

1 **ACTION**

CLEAR THE AIRWAY — Make sure that nothing is obstructing the air flow from the mouth and throat through to the lungs.
See page 10.

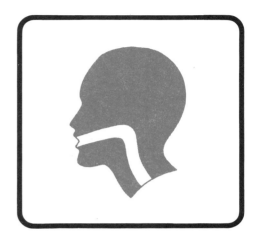

2 ENSURE AIR FLOW TO LUNGS — Begin artificial ventilation without delay — seconds count.
See page 10.

3 RESTART THE HEARTBEAT — If no pulse can be felt, by artificially pumping the heart if necessary.
See page 12.

Asthma

IMPORTANT

Asthma occurs commonly in childhood and is due to exertion, emotion, allergy or infection or a combination of all three.
Symptoms: Sudden attack of tight, difficult breathing — often occurring at night; difficulty in forcing air *out* of lungs; anxiety; pale and clammy skin; rapid pulse; blueness around lips.

Common causes of asthma due to allergies are feathers, house dust, pollens and milk products

1 Sit or prop child up comfortably — leaning forward and resting on a table, pillow or back of a chair — but keep back straight.

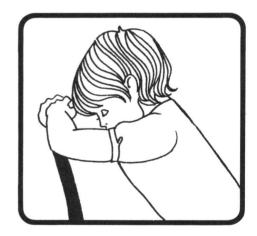

2 Calm and reassure the child and ensure quiet surroundings. Allow plenty of fresh air — cigarette smoke, dust and cooking smells can make it worse.

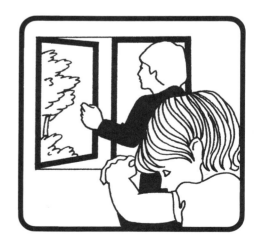

38

Asthma

3 Give hot drinks to ease the tension.

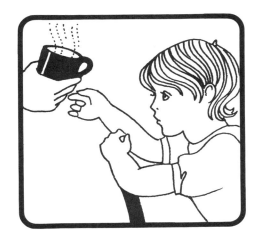

4 Assist with asthma using relieving drugs, if these are present and the dose is known.

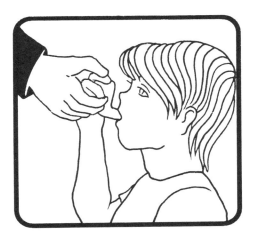

5 Summon medical help if severity of attack demands.
Watch the breathing: if it stops give artificial ventilation —
see page 10.
Check the pulse: if it stops apply heart compression – see page 12.

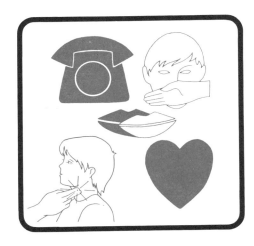

Bites & stings

IMPORTANT

If the skin has been penetrated, seek immediate medical advice.

Do not underestimate the severity of human bites — they can be particularly dangerous.

In countries where *rabies* may be present, all children bitten by dogs should be referred for special serum treatment. Try to capture or confine the offending animal for examination

1 Calm, reassure and lay the child down. Wash the wound well with soap and water. Gently dry. Do not apply antiseptic creams and ointments.

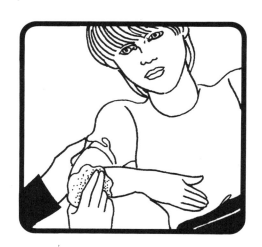

2 Cover with sterile gauze or a clean cloth and hold in place with adhesive tape or bandage.

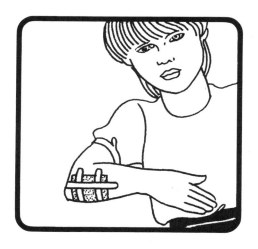

Watch for shock — see page 116 for treatment

Bites & stings

BEDBUGS, SAND FLIES & MOSQUITOES

Symptoms: Vary from itchy red spots to mildly painful swellings.

Seek medical advice if child suffers an allergic reaction to any insect bites

1 Wash the affected area with soap and water. Apply cold compresses if swellings are present.

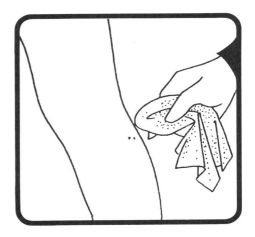

2 Apply calamine lotion, cologne or cheap perfume. Use antihistamine tablets if the bites are very itchy.

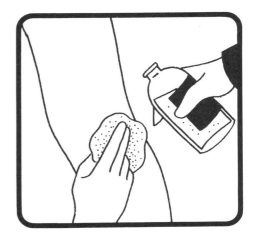

Bites & stings

Some children have an allergic reaction to bee and wasp stings. Seek medical advice if symptoms are severe

BEES, HORNETS, WASPS & YELLOW JACKETS

Symptoms: Sudden pricking pain which may become severe, local swelling, burning and itching.

1 Remove sting (if present) by scraping with the back of a knife or a plastic card.

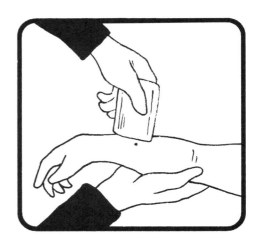

2 Do not squeeze or rub the skin.

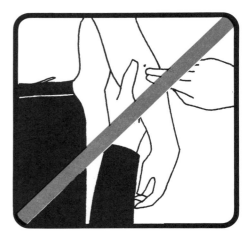

Bites & stings

3 Apply cold compress for pain relief. Be alert in case of allergic reaction.

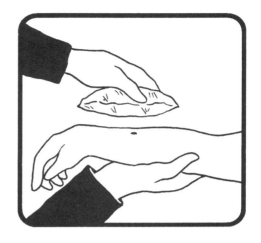

4 If the sting is in or around the mouth, swelling can result in airway obstruction. URGENT medial care is required. Call an ambulance.

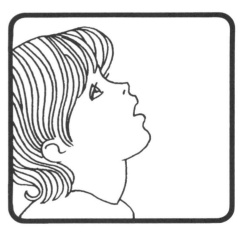

5 Watch for signs of shock and, if necessary give the treatment described on page 116. Watch the breathing: if it stops give artificial ventilation — see page 10.

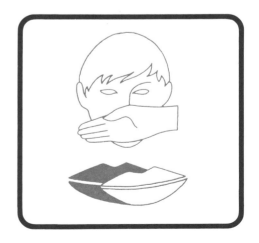

Bites & stings

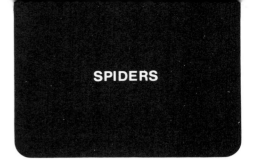
REDBACK, FUNNELWEB & ALL SNAKES

Symptoms: Pain at bite site, tingling around mouth, profuse sweating, drooling, abdominal pain, nausea and sometimes breathing difficulty.
Follow procedure below and transport child to hospital immediately.

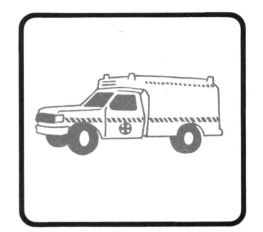

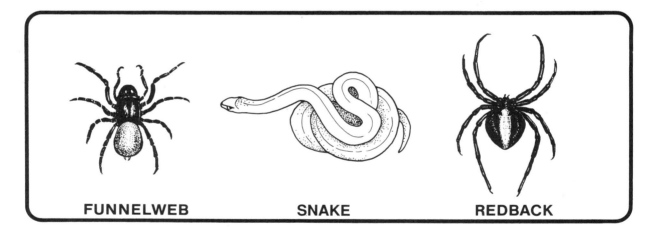

| FUNNELWEB | SNAKE | REDBACK |

1 Calm and reassure the child and keep under constant observation. For redback spider bites: the bite sight becomes hot, red and swollen with intense local pain. Apply a cold compress to reduce pain and transport the child to hospital by ambulance.

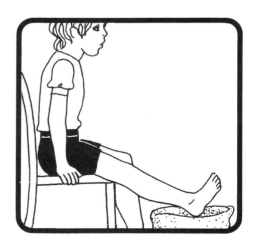

Bites & stings

2 For funnelweb bites: apply firm local pressure over the bite site. Firmly apply a crepe bandage around the limb, over the area of the bite. Then bandage from the bite to the fingers or toes then upwards to cover as much of the limb as possible. Apply as tightly as for a sprained ankle. The bandage may be applied over clothing.

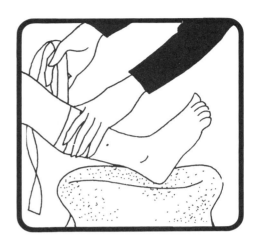

3 Splint the limb to immobilise it completely. Transport the child to hospital, moving him, and particularly the bitten limb, as little as possible.

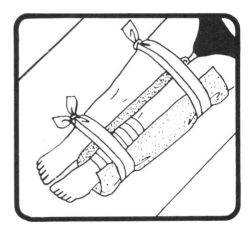

4 Watch the breathing: if it stops give artificial ventilation — see page 10.
Check the pulse: if it stops apply heart compression – see page 12.
Watch for signs of shock and, if necessary give the treatment described on page 116.

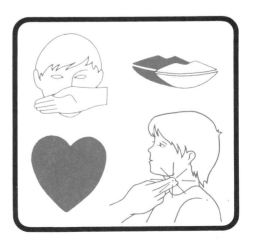

Bites & stings

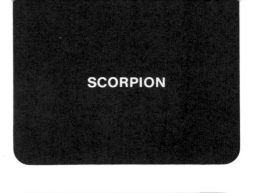

SCORPION

Seek immediate medical advice.

Symptoms: Severe pain at site of sting. Swelling, fever, nausea and stomach pains. Difficulty in speaking, convulsions and coma.

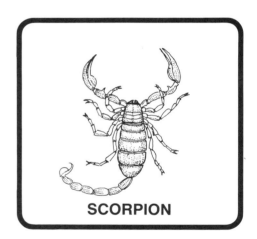

SCORPION

Treat as for spider bites on previous pages and again check breathing and pulse.

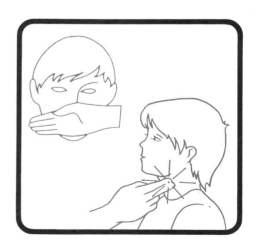

Bites & stings

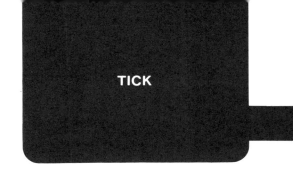

Symptoms: Pin prick and irritation. The tick may be visible on the skin. Ticks, which are most active in Spring and Summer, rarely cause paralysis in humans.

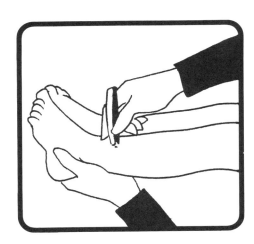

TICK

1 By levering out, make sure that the head does not remain under the skin.

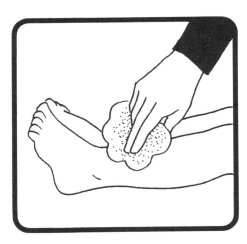

2 Wash with soap and water.

Bites & stings

CONE SHELL & SEA URCHIN

Symptoms: Vary from slight sting to severe pain, tingling and numbness, difficulty in swallowing, tightness in the chest, partial paralysis, blurring of vision and collapse.

A Marine Stinger Hotline is available 24 hours for urgent advice on marine information. The number is toll free 008 079 909.

1 Calm and reassure the child. Carry to safety and comfort. If the sting is on the arm or leg, treat as for funnelweb bite — see page 44/45.

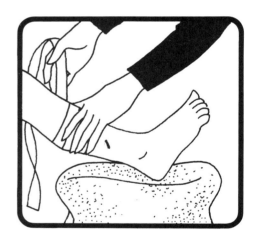

2 Transport to hospital by ambulance, moving the child and particularly the affected limb as little as possible. Keep the child under constant observation.

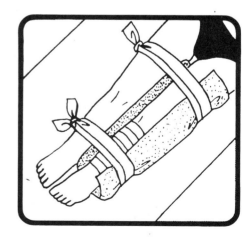

Bites & stings

JELLYFISH & BLUE BOTTLE

Signs & symptoms: These include — skin pain, wheals, pain in groin and armpits, nausea, headache, vomiting and breathing difficulty. However, these signs & symptoms may vary in individual cases.

ACTION: If sting is from a large jellyfish apply cold compress and treat as for a funnelweb bite (page 45). Anti-venom is available for box jellyfish. Apply cold compress soaked in soluble aspirin if itchy or irritated and give antihistamine tablets.

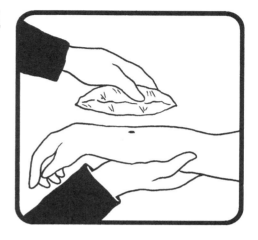

SEA ANEMONE & HYDROID

Symptoms: Same as for jellyfish and blue bottle.

ACTION: As for blue bottle stings. If cold compress is not available, quickly remove remaining tentacles by pinching off with fingers and applying pressure. Apply immobilisation bandage to the limb including the sting area.

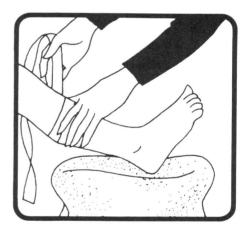

Watch the breathing: if it stops, give artificial ventilation — see page 10
Check the pulse: if it stops apply heart compression — see page 12. Watch for signs of shock and, if necessary give the treatment described on page 116.

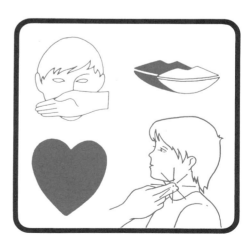

Bites & stings

Seek immediate medical advice.

STINGING CORAL

Symptoms: Local burning or stinging pain.

ACTION: As for blue bottle stings — see page 49.

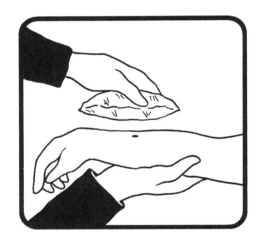

STINGRAY

Symptoms: Sudden pain, swelling and redness around wound; nausea and vomiting. Sometimes muscle spasms, convulsions and breathing difficulties.

1 Carefully remove the stinger if possible.

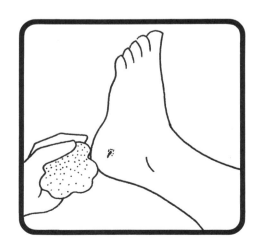

Bites & stings

2 Control bleeding if necessary (see page 54). Otherwise treat as for spider bites (see page 44).

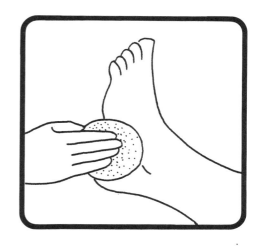

3 Watch the breathing: if it stops give artificial ventilation — see page 10.
Check the pulse: if it stops apply heart compression – see page 12.
Watch for signs of shock and, if necessary give the treatment described on page 116.

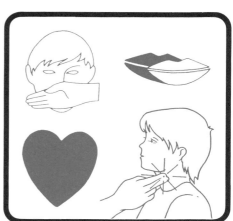

BLUE-RINGED OCTOPUS

Symptoms: Weakness of the muscles and numbness, breathing becomes progressively more difficult. As soon as this happens begin artificial ventilation (see page 10) and maintain until medical aid arrives.

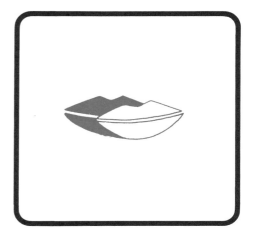

Bites & stings

IMPORTANT

In all cases of snakebite, especially if the snake is known to be poisonous, seek immediate medical attention.
Symptoms: Headache, nausea and vomiting, weakness, blurring of vision and difficulty in speaking, swallowing and breathing. These effects are not usually seen for hours. However, in cases of massive impregnation of venom signs and symptoms may appear within minutes.

1 Calm, reassure and lay the child down. Move the affected part as little as possible.

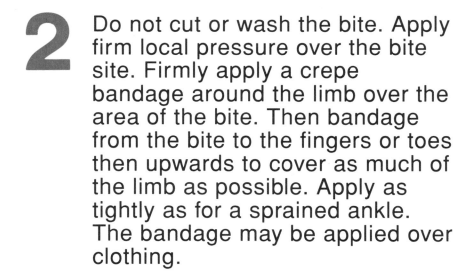

2 Do not cut or wash the bite. Apply firm local pressure over the bite site. Firmly apply a crepe bandage around the limb over the area of the bite. Then bandage from the bite to the fingers or toes then upwards to cover as much of the limb as possible. Apply as tightly as for a sprained ankle. The bandage may be applied over clothing.

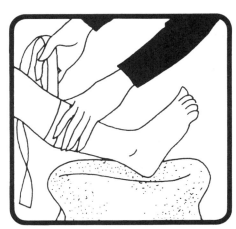

Serious poisoning is comparatively rare in man because significant quantities of venom are seldom injected

Bites & stings

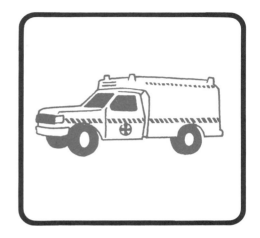

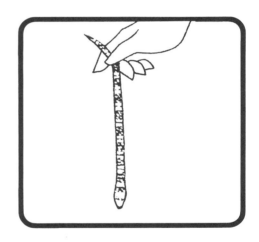

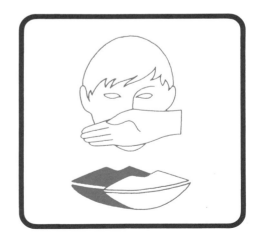

SNAKE BITES

3 Splint the limb to immobilise it completely. Transport the child to the nearest medical aid, moving the bitten limb as little as possible.

4 Great caution should be taken to prevent further bites. If the snake is dead, bring it to the hospital. Handle by the tail and place in a bag or sack.

5 Watch the breathing: if it stops give artificial ventilation — see page 10.
Watch for signs of shock and, if necessary give the treatment described on page 116.

Fear of death is a common reaction to snakebite and tends to accelerate the effect of the venom

Bleeding

IMPORTANT

Any bleeding can look alarming — it is nature's way of shouting for help — but bleeding from a small wound will usually stop of its own accord after about 30 seconds and can be easily controlled by local pressure. Abrasions and minor cuts are best left open to the air and kept dry, unless they occur beneath clothing.

Send for medical help only if the bleeding cannot be stopped within a few minutes

1 Rest, comfort and reassure the child.

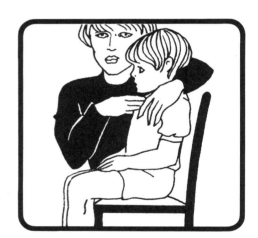

2 If the wound is dirty, gently wash for a few seconds in running water.

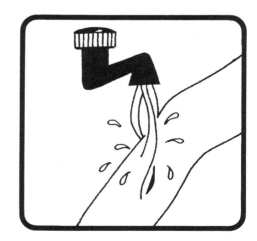

Bleeding

3 Press clean gauze or cloth directly over wound and dry the surrounding area if previously bathed.

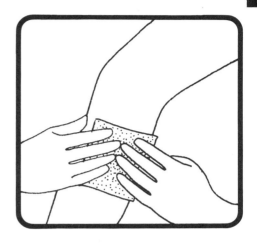

4 Replace soaked gauze with a clean dressing and attach with adhesive plaster or bandage.

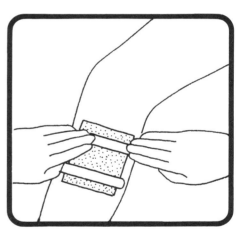

5 Elevate and support the injured part above heart level.

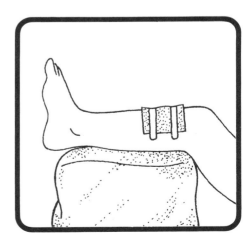

Bleeding

Aim to stop the bleeding and obtain medical help at once. Move the child as little as possible, especially if an underlying fracture is suspected.

Symptoms: Where much blood has been lost, the face and lips become pale, the skin is cold and clammy, the child feels faint or dizzy, can become restless, thirsty, sick and has a rapid, weak pulse with shallow breathing.

1 Lay the child down and give comfort and reassurance. Immediately apply direct pressure over the bleeding area with whatever clean tissue comes to hand, for 5 to 15 minutes.

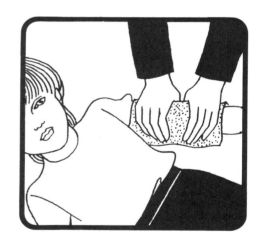

2 Raise and support the injured part, unless an underlying fracture is suspected. Any visible foreign bodies that can be picked out or wiped off should be removed. Do not remove impaled objects.

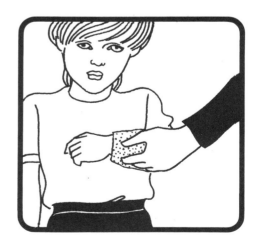

Do not give drinks — sips only — as the child may need an anaesthetic before wound is stitched

56

Bleeding

3 Apply a clean dressing and press this firmly over the wound. Cover this with a pad of soft material and retain in place with firm bandaging. Make sure the whole wound is covered. If bleeding continues, apply further firm dressings and bandage over the original.

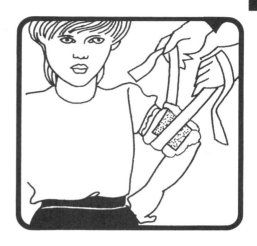

4 Immobilise an arm in a sling, or a leg by tying to its fellow with adequate padding.

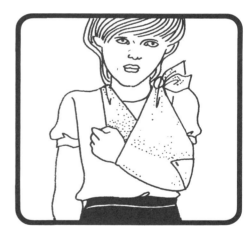

5 Watch the breathing: if it stops give emergency resuscitation – see page 10.
Check the pulse: if it stops apply heart compression – see page 12.
Watch for signs of shock and, if necessary give the treatment described on page 116.

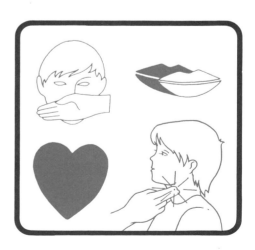

Virtually all bleeding can be stopped by pressure upon the wound. Tourniquets are dangerous and should not be used

Bleeding

If internal bleeding is suspected, summon immediate medical aid. Internal bleeding may be suspected if a child has a broken bone or has sustained a sharp blow, knife or bullet wound to the head, chest or abdomen.

Symptoms vary according to the location of the bleeding:

* HEAD: Severe headache, dizziness, vomiting, double vision, loss of consciousness.
* CHEST: Bright red foamy blood is coughed up.
* STOMACH: Bright, dark or 'coffee-grounds' coloured vomit.
* INTESTINES: Black tar-coloured stools.
* SPLEEN, LIVER: No visible bleeding: child becomes rapidly shocked and may have stomach pain.

Internal bleeding can also occur as a result of certain medical conditions. If in doubt consult your doctor immediately

1 Place child at complete rest with legs slightly raised and loosen any tight clothing. Calm and reassure the child.

Look for other injuries and treat as necessary.

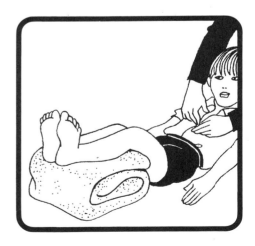

Do NOT remove any impaled objects.

58

Bleeding

2 Protect from cold.

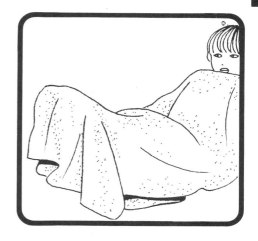

3 Give nothing to drink.

4 Watch the breathing: if it stops give artificial ventilation — see page 10.
Check the pulse: if it stops apply heart compression — see page 12. Seek medical assistance.

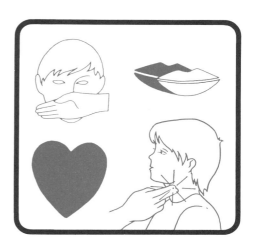

Bleeding

IMPORTANT

Bleeding from the nose is very common and does not usually denote anything serious. It is usually due to a ruptured blood vessel in the *septum* which divides the nostrils. However, it is possible that severe head injuries may cause blood to trickle from the nose.

Seek immediate medical advice if a fracture is suspected

1 Place the child in a sitting position with head slightly forward.

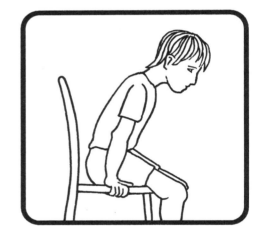

2 Tell him to pinch firmly the soft part of his nose for about 10 minutes and to breathe through his mouth.

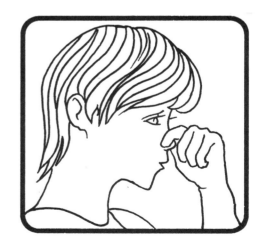

Bleeding

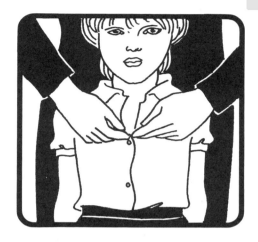

3 Loosen any tight clothing.

4 Apply a cold compress over forehead and bridge of nose. Warn the child not to blow his nose for some hours and not to pick it.

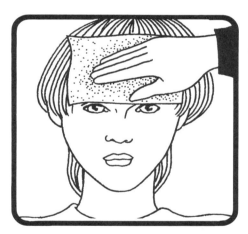

5 If bleeding is not controlled or recommences when the pressure is removed, seek prompt medical aid.

Burns & scalds

IMPORTANT

Take the child to hospital immediately if the burn is more than very slight. Burns may be **deep** or **superficial**: deep burns usually destroy nerve endings and are least painful; superficial burns, involving only the outer layers of skin, are most painful and can result in considerable fluid loss.

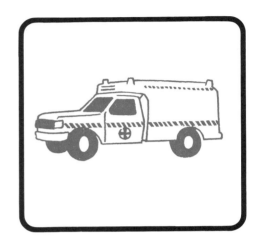

1 Gently flood the affected area immediately with cold water (not ice). Continue for 10 minutes or until the pain stops. Do not apply pressure over burned skin, or try to remove nylon clothing which has become stuck to the skin.

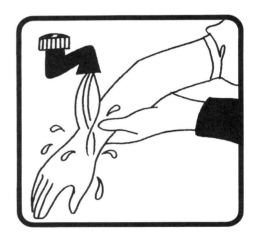

2 Remove promptly any tight clothing over the area, such as rings, bangles, belts and shoes. Carefully remove any clothing which has been soaked in boiling water. Do not try to remove damaged tissue or break blisters, or remove any clothing which is stuck to the wound.

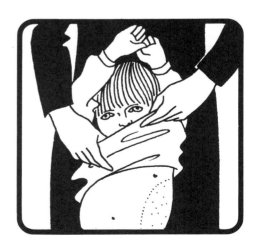

Burns & scalds

3 Cover loosely with a clean dry dressing, such as gauze, handkerchief, pillow case or strip of sheet. Elevate and support injured arms or legs higher than the chest. Do not apply any home remedies such as ointments and antiseptic creams.

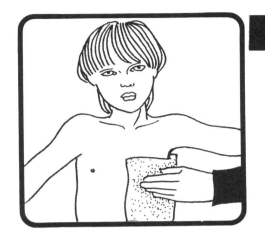

4 Give frequent small cold drinks if burns are bad. This will help to replace fluid loss.

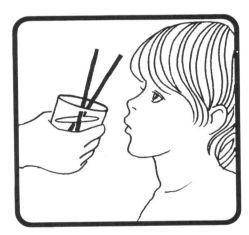

5 Watch the breathing: if it stops give artificial ventilation — see page 10.

Watch for signs of shock and, if necessary give the treatment described on page 116.

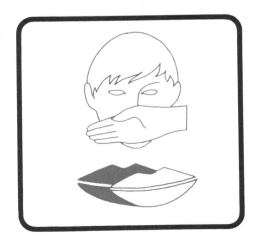

Chest injuries

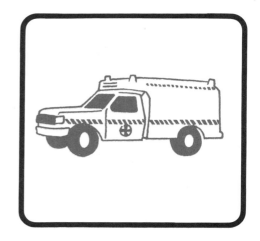

IMPORTANT

If any severe injury to chest, or fracture to rib(s) is suspected take the child to hospital immediately. Symptoms may include pain in chest on breathing and severe pain on touching the injured area. The chest may collapse rather than expand on inhaling. There may be difficulty in breathing and shock.

1 If one or two broken ribs are suspected, gently but firmly and not too tightly bind the arm on the injured side across the chest — to help immobilise injury.

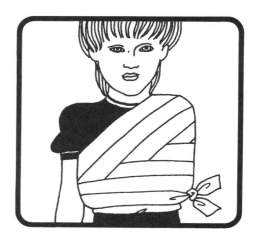

2 If the injury is more severe and breathing is difficult, lay child down with head and shoulders raised and body inclined toward the injured side.

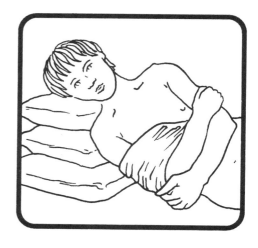

Chest injuries

3 Loosen all tight clothing.

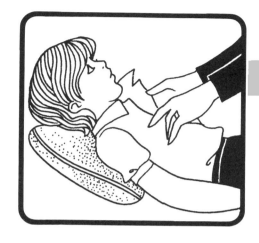

4 Facilitate fresh air, peace and calm — to reduce breathing effort.

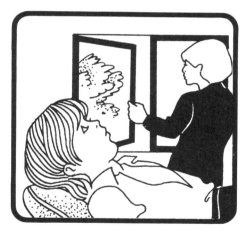

5 Watch the breathing: if it stops give artificial ventilation — see page 10.
Check the pulse: if it stops apply heart compression – see page 12.
Watch for signs of shock and if necessary give the treatment described on page 116.

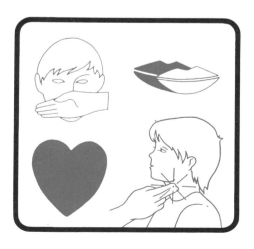

Chest injuries

IMPORTANT

For all penetrating wounds seek immediate medical help.
Symptoms: There will be pain associated with breathing and there is a danger that air is sucked into the chest cavity through the wound. Blood or blood-stained bubbles may ooze from wound and the child may cough up bright red, frothy blood.

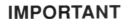

1 Place the palm of the hand firmly and quickly over the wound until a dressing can be applied. The main aim is to seal the wound immediately and so prevent air entering the chest cavity.

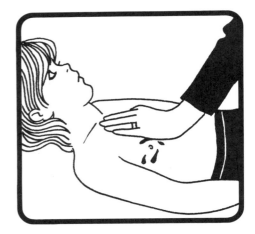

2 Cover with a non-porous dressing (ie: plastic, foil etc) and seal on three sides leaving the bottom edge free.

IMPORTANT

Do not remove impaled objects. The only exception to this is in a cardiac arrest situation with an impaled object in the chest where removal is necessary to facilitate CPR.

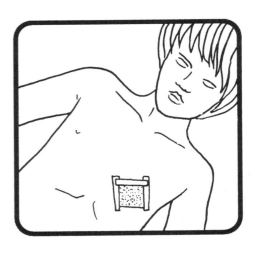

66

Chest injuries

3 Lay the child down with head and shoulders raised and the body inclined towards injured side.

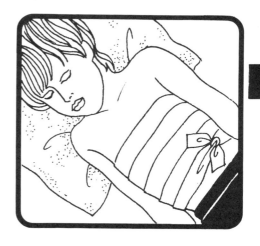

4 Loosen any tight clothing and provide fresh air and calm surroundings.

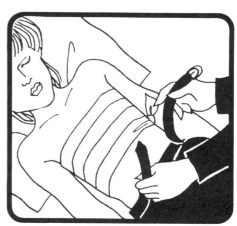

5 Keep the airway clear, see page 10.
Watch the breathing: if it stops give artificial ventilation —
see page 10.
Watch for signs of shock and, if necessary give the treatment described on page 116.

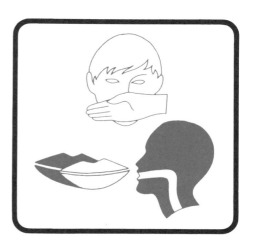

Choking

IMPORTANT

If choking persists or congestion becomes apparent, summon immediate medical attention.

Symptoms: Usually the first symptom is a sudden fit of coughing, the face and neck may become red turning to purple. There may be violent and alarming attempts by the child to get his breath.

1 Remove obvious obstruction; eg food, toy or nut but do not interfere with the child's own efforts to clear the obstruction.

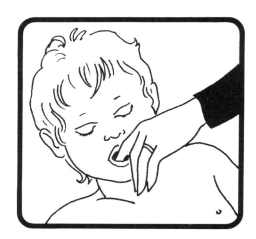

2 ## INFANTS

Lay infant along arm or leg with head inclined down and give up to four back blows between the shoulders — repeat again if unsuccessful.

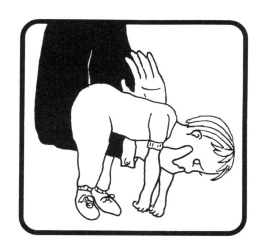

Choking

3 **OLDER CHILDREN**
Lay child over your knees with head down and give up to four back blows between the shoulders — repeat if unsuccessful.

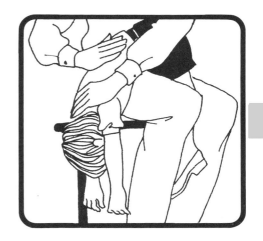

4 **IF CHOKING CONTINUES**
Persist with airway clearance until medical aid arrives. Back blows may be used in the unconscious or non breathing child.

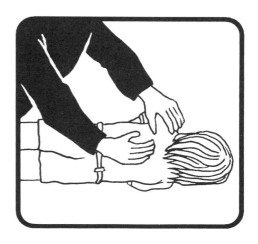

5 Watch the breathing: if it stops give artificial ventilation — see page 10.

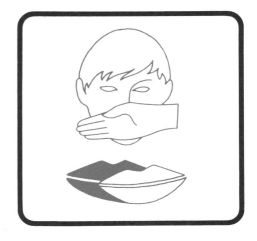

69

Convulsions

IMPORTANT

The child may fall to the ground, stiffen the whole body which may arch backwards, froth at the mouth, begin uncontrollable jerking movements and may be unconscious when the shaking is over. There may be a high temperature.

Do not try to restrain the child and offer nothing to drink during the attack

1 Clear the surroundings of hard or sharp objects that could cause harm.

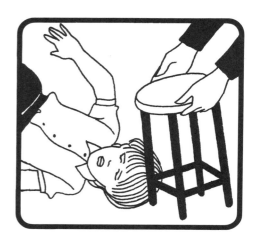

2 Loosen any tight clothing, especially around the neck, chest or waist. Place nothing in the mouth during the fit, including your fingers. It is impossible for anyone to swallow their tongue.

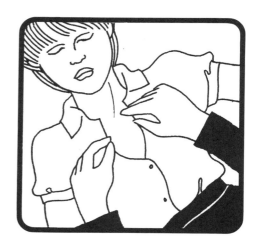

Convulsions

3 When the convulsion has stopped lift the child onto a soft chair, settee or bed and lay him on one side without a pillow. Cover with a warm blanket or coat if cold.

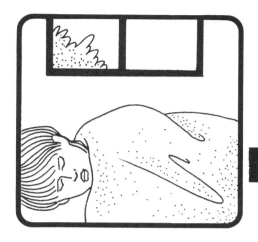

4 If the child is hot, remove excess clothing or covers and wipe with a tepid sponge. Do not put child in a bath in case he or she fits again.

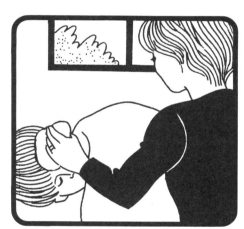

5 Watch the breathing: if it stops give artificial ventilation — see page 10. Remove to hospital by ambulance.

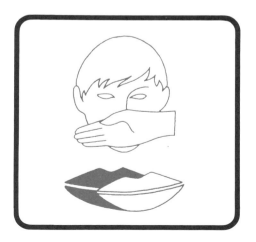

Cramp

Symptoms: Sudden painful tight muscle or group of muscles. Cramp commonly occurs while exercising in cold; eg swimming, or during exertion in hot conditions where a lot of sweating takes place.

In sports and games, pulled muscles may be confused with cramp. Do not stretch muscles or straighten limbs without the aid of massage

1 Forcibly but gently stretch the stiffened part until straight. Firmly rub and massage the affected muscle with your warm hands, until cramp eases.

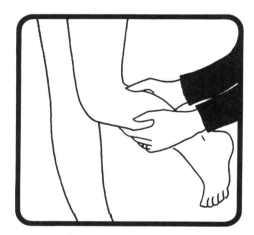

2 When there has been much sweating, and therefore much salt and water loss, give plenty of water to drink in which salt has been added: half teaspoonful salt to one large glass of water.

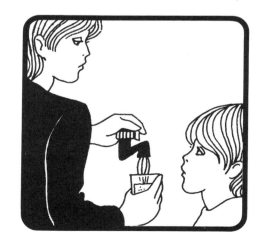

Drowning

IMPORTANT

Send for immediate medical aid. Fresh water in the lungs is largely absorbed. Sea water is less well absorbed and more dangerous. Sometimes spasms of the voice-box will prevent water entering lungs.

1 On arrival on land immediately hold child hanging over your knee for 5 to 10 seconds to encourage free drainage of water from airway. If necessary, commence resuscitation at once.

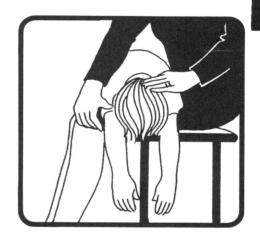

2 If the child is unconscious and not breathing, begin immediate resuscitation, in the water if necessary. See page 10.

Any child having suffered a near drowning must be taken to hospital as complications may take some hours to occur.

73

Ear injuries

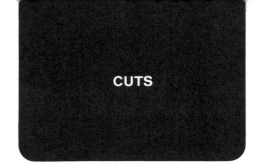

Ear injuries are commonly due to cuts, foreign bodies and infection. Occasionally they may be associated with severe head injuries. If such injuries are suspected, seek immediate medical aid.

1 Control bleeding from cuts by pressing gauze or a clean cloth directly over the wound and elevate the child's head.

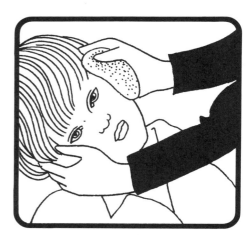

2 Hold the gauze in place with a bandage around the child's head.

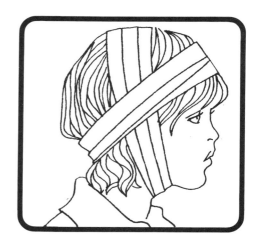

74

Ear injuries

Seek medical aid in the event of foreign bodies proving to be immoveable, and in cases of infection.

Foreign bodies: Insects may be removed by gently flooding the ear with tepid water or olive oil. If the insect is alive it may be attracted from the ear by a lighted candle held 15cm away. Beads, beans, nuts and other solid objects should be removed by a doctor.

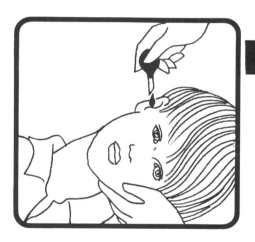

Infection: Bleeding and pus from the ear usually indicates infection and possibly perforation of the ear drum. Place a wad of cotton wool loosely in the ear and hold in place with a bandage.

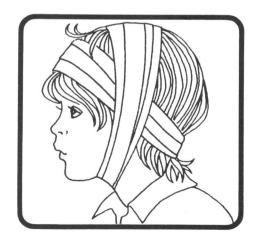

Electric shock

IMPORTANT

Injuries due to electric shock from low voltage contact are not usually severe, but may be more serious if the child is very young. Clinical shock (see page 116) is a likely consequence.

Avoid direct contact with child while he is in contact with the current

1 Break the contact by switching off the current, removing the plug or wrenching the cable free.

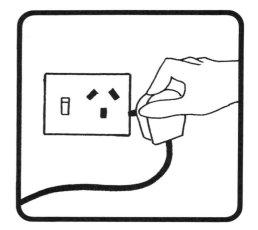

2 If the above action is not possible, stand on something dry (blanket, rubber mat, newspapers) and break the contact by pushing the child free with a wooden pole or board, or pulling with a loop of rope around an arm or leg.

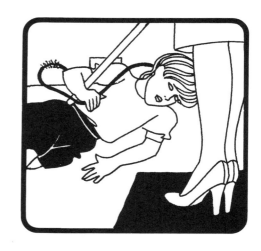

If necessary, treat the child for heat burns. See page 62

76

Electric shock

IMPORTANT

Injuries due to high voltage contact may be very severe — even fatal — involving burns to the skin and possibly to internal organs.
High voltage electricity is usually carried by overhead cables or conductor rails. When a main power supply is involved, contact the police immediately.

Never attempt rescue while the child is in contact with the current. Keep others away from the casualty

1 Only assist with First Aid when you are told officially that it is safe to do so — ie when the current has been switched off.

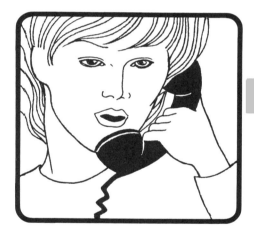

2 If the child is apparently dead, resuscitation is the first priority. See page 10.

77

Eye injuries

IMPORTANT

All eye injuries are potentially serious and will require medical attention.

Do not attempt to remove a foreign body which is on the pupil of the eye. Prevent the child rubbing the eye

1 Remove the foreign body from white of eye with the corner of a clean handkerchief or a moistened wisp of cotton wool. If under the lower lid, pull the lid down and remove foreign body as shown.

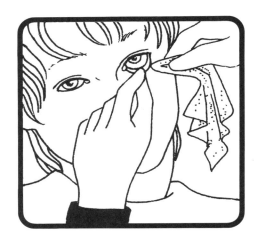

2 If this is unsuccessful or the object is under the upper lid, ask the child to blink with the eye under water.

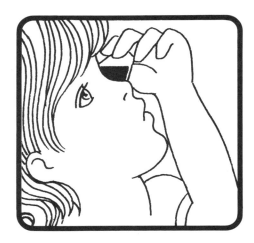

Eye injuries

CHEMICALS IN EYE

Holding the eyelid open, gently run tepid water over the eye for 15 minutes.

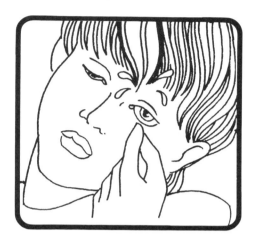

PENETRATING INJURIES

Lay the child down and give comfort and reassurance. Cover only the injured eye with gauze padding held in place with a light bandage around the head.

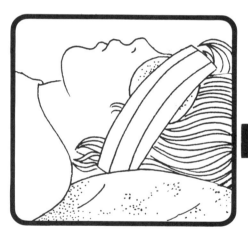

Transport to hospital immediately by ambulance.

Exposure

IMPORTANT

Hypothermia is a dangerous condition in which the central part of the body cools below normal.
Symptoms: The child is usually quiet and refuses food and drinks, he is sluggish, and may be drowsy. The skin may be deceptively pink but is cold. The pulse is slow and weak. The breathing can be slow and shallow.

Do not use hot water bottles or electric blankets which could well heat the body too quickly and dangerously lower the blood pressure

1 Prevent further heat loss by removing the child from cold conditions and giving shelter.

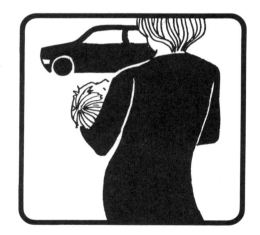

2 Gradually warm the child by placing between warm blankets and/or cuddling him against your own body.

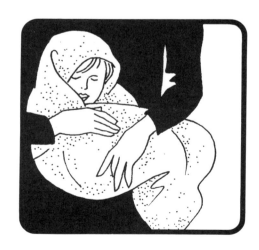

Infants are especially susceptible to exposure because their body temperature regulating mechanisms are not yet fully efficient

80

Exposure

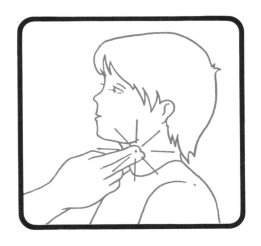

HYPOTHERMIA

3 Take the pulse at regular intervals.

4 If the child is conscious, give tepid or warm sweet drinks.

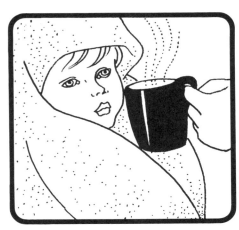

5 If the condition does not improve in about ½ hour summon medical help.

Fever

IMPORTANT

Take the child's temperature (see page 18) before deciding on your course of action.

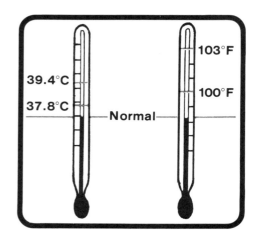

1 If the temperature is below 37.8°C (100°F) simply remove any excess clothing or bed covers. Cold drinks — fruit juice (not squash) milk or water — can be offered.

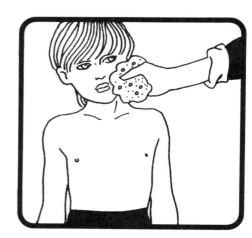

2 If temperature is above 37.8°C (100°F) and especially if it is above 39.4°C (103°F), place tepid cloths around the neck and in the armpits and groin. Continue to sponge the body with tepid water until temperature is reduced. Paracetamol will rapidly reduce high temperatures. Your local hospital or poisons information centre will advise you what doses are suitable for your child. Larger than normal doses may be required.

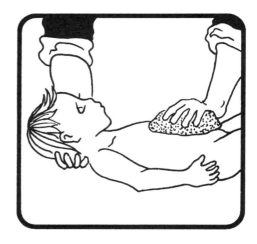

82

Fever

3 Dry the child well and cover only in light clothing or a sheet.

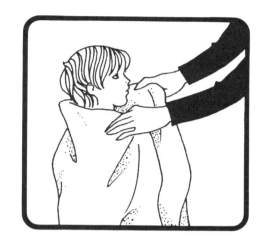

4 Keep in a cool (but not cold) room and give cold drinks. In the tropics, drinks should be salty.

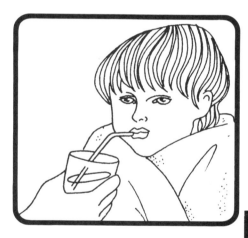

5 Keep in a cool (but not cold) room and check the temperature every half hour. If the temperature remains above 39.4°C (103°F) for more than one hour or if the child is obviously distressed, seek medical advice.

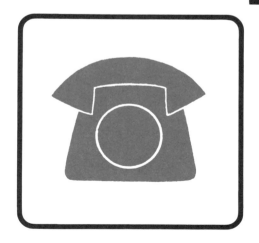

Fractures

Every child with a definite or suspected fracture or dislocation should receive medical attention as soon as possible. Transport of the child should be as gentle as possible.

Fractures are often difficult to diagnose in a child. If in doubt, treat as a fracture of bone or dislocation of joint. Most fractures in children are incomplete and are called 'greenstick' fractures, (*see diagram*).

Symptoms of fractures and dislocations may vary considerably but will include one or more of the following:

Pain at or near the site of injury made worse by movement of the part.

Tenderness when gentle pressure is applied to affected part.

Swelling due to blood loss around fracture.

Loss of control – deformity of limb, inability to move, or unnatural movement of, injured part.

Coarse bony grating of broken ends of fractured bone — uncommon in young children.

Shock due to blood loss — internal or external.

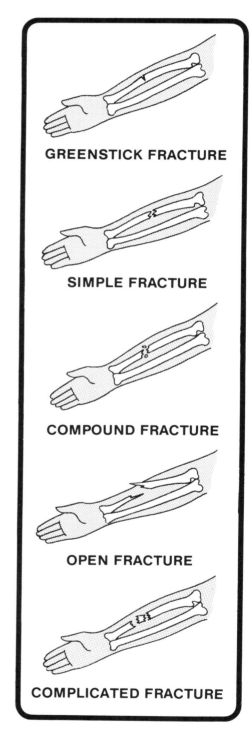

GREENSTICK FRACTURE

SIMPLE FRACTURE

COMPOUND FRACTURE

OPEN FRACTURE

COMPLICATED FRACTURE

Fractures

1 Attend to asphyxia (see page 36), bleeding and severe wounds before dealing with fracture.

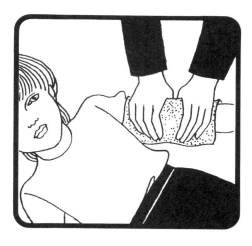

2 Move child as little as possible from site of accident — move only if life (child's or your own) is endangered. Move child by pulling him along, holding him underneath the armpits.

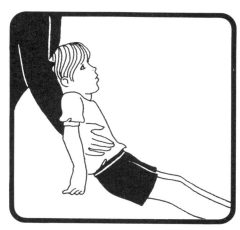

3 Immobilise part as soon as possible and in any case before moving the child too far, using the child's body and bandages as means of support or using splints and bandages. Raise the injured part after immobilisation to reduce pain and swelling.

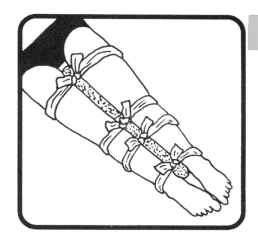

Fractures

IMPORTANT

Every child with a definite or suspected fracture or dislocation should receive medical attention as soon as possible. Transport of the child should be as gentle as possible. Care in use of bandages is essential — they must be tight enough to immobilise the part but not so tight as to interfere with the circulation.

1 Separate skin surfaces with soft padding before bandaging — this avoids chafing of skin. Tie knots over a splint or on the uninjured side.

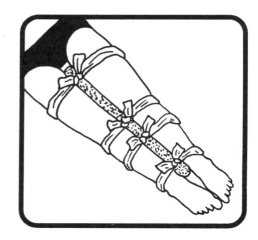

2 Check the tightness of bandaging every 10 minutes because of swelling — especially important in elbow injuries — loosen slightly when necessary.

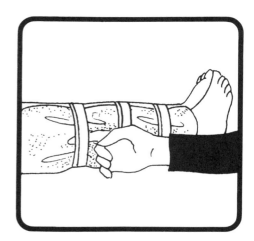

Fractures

Splints if and when used should be:

Sufficiently rigid and long enough to immobilise the joint above and the joint below a fracture.

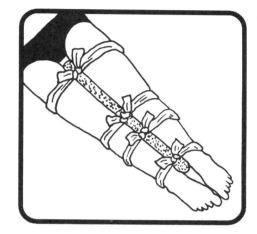

They must also be well padded, wide enough to immobilise the part and should be applied over clothing.

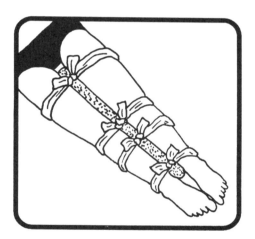

Splints may be improvised from walking sticks, umbrellas, broom handles, pieces of wood, cardboard or firmly folded newspapers or magazines.

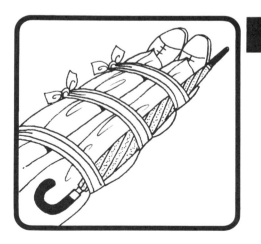

87

Fractures

Move the child as little as possible to avoid damage to the spinal cord. Comfort the child and encourage him to lie still at all times. Give only sips of fluid, in case unconsciousness should occur. Remove to hospital as soon as possible and watch for shock.

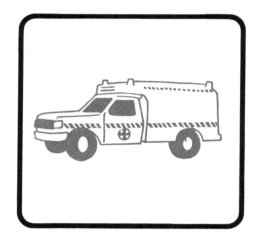

1 If medical help is readily available, do as little as possible. Child should be lying down on flat, firm surface.

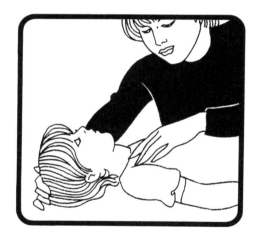

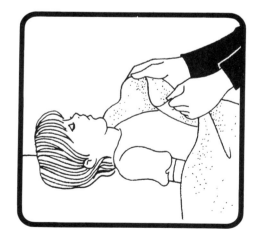

2 Instruct the child to lie still. Cover with a blanket and await the arrival of medical help.

88

Fractures

3 If you need to transport the child to medical help, seek help in preparing the casualty. Devise a stretcher out of a sturdy board, door etc. Place the board, covered with a blanket, next to the child who should have been turned onto his side facing away from the stretcher.

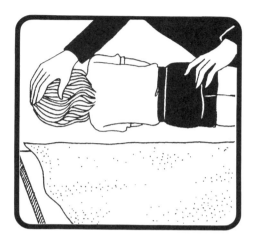

4 Do not twist the child during placing onto stretcher. Move his body as single unit, keeping the head in line with the spine. On a signal from the person holding the head, roll and lift the child gently onto the stretcher without twisting the body or head.

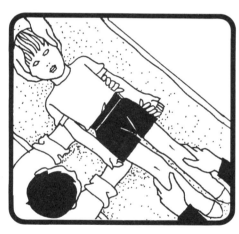

5 Immobilise the head and spine with suitable padding and bind to stretcher with bandages, belts, scarves, etc.

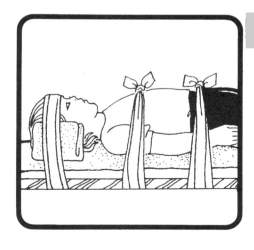

Fractures

Remove child to hospital as soon as possible. Meanwhile watch for shock.

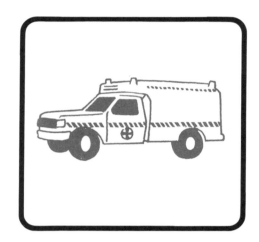

COLLARBONE, SHOULDER OR BENT ELBOW

Support the weight of the arm in a sling made from a triangular bandage. Immobilise the arm by gently tying a band over the sling and around the body.

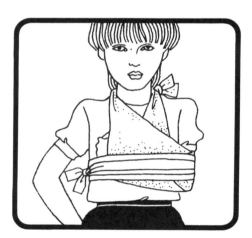

STRAIGHT ELBOW

1 Do not attempt to bend elbow. Lay the child down and place the injured arm gently by child's side, palm to thigh.

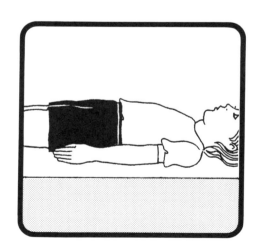

Fractures

2 Place adequate soft padding between the arm and the side of the body.

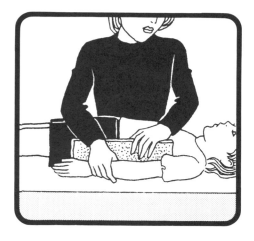

3 Secure broad bandages around the arm and body, tied on the uninjured side of the body.

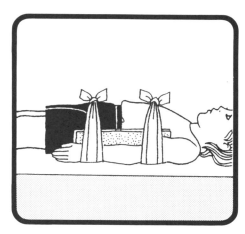

4 Transport on a stretcher.

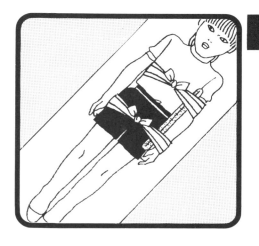

Fractures

Remove child to hospital as soon as possible and watch for shock.

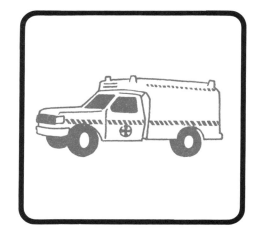

1 Immobilise lower arm with padded splint — do not tie too tightly.

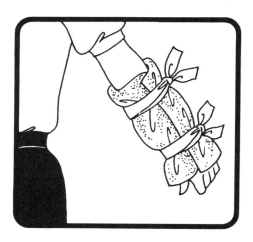

2 Support the weight of the arm in a sling made from a folded scarf or a triangular bandage. Secure the arm to the chest by a broad bandage applied over the sling.

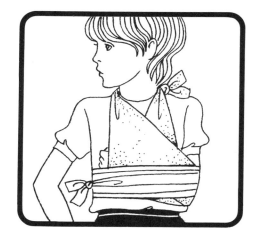

Fractures

1 Lay the child down flat on back with legs straight. If the child wishes to bend his knees slightly, they should be supported on a folded blanket.

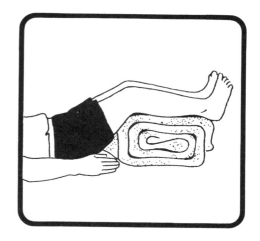

2 Place thick padding between the thighs and secure broad bandages around the pelvis, knees and ankles.

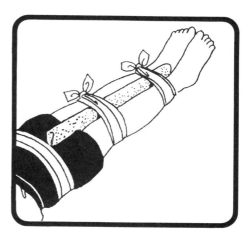

3 Transport on a stretcher.

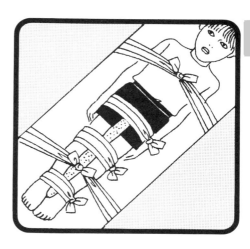

Fractures

Remove child to hospital as soon as possible. Meanwhile, watch for shock.

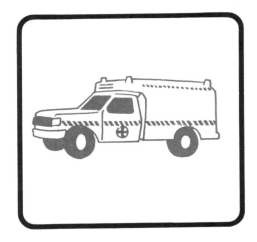

1 Immobilise the injured leg in the position found using padded splints. If the knee is straight, extend the splint from the buttock to the heel.

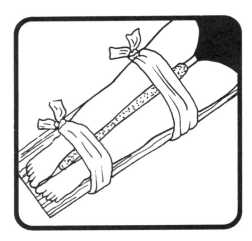

2 Transport by stretcher.

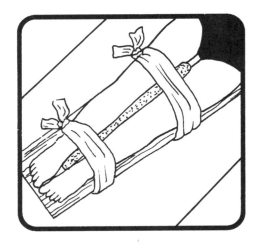

Fractures

1 Lay the child flat, with head and shoulders propped up. Lay the injured leg alongside the straightened normal leg.

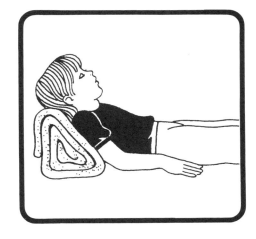

2 Immobilise with a padded splint. If it is impossible to improvise a splint, place padding between the legs and tie them together.

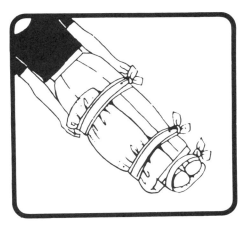

3 Transport by stretcher.

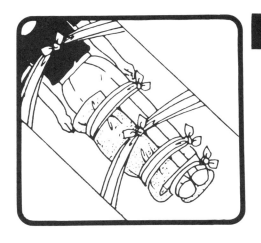

Fractures

Remove child to hospital as soon as possible. Meanwhile watch for shock.

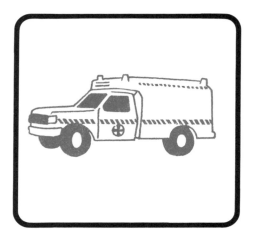

1 Carefully remove the shoe or boot and sock or stocking, cutting if necessary.

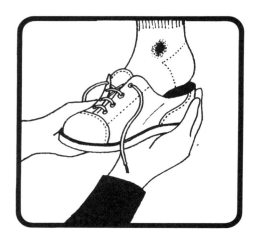

2 Treat any wounds which may be present (see page 54).

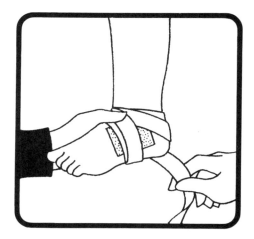

Fractures

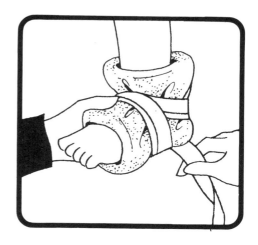

3 Tie a well -padded support around foot.

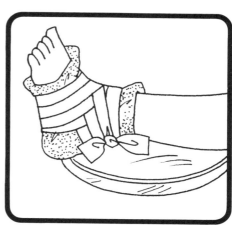

4 Support the leg and foot on a pillow, or rolled-up blanket or overcoat.

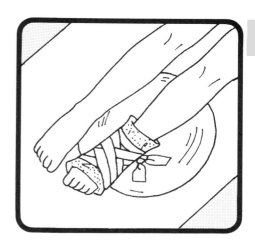

5 Transport by stretcher.

Frostbite

Frostbite occurs when part of the body is exposed for any length of time to the wind in very cold weather. The ears, nose, chin, fingers and toes are most frequently affected.
Symptoms: The affected part feels cold, numb, painful and stiff. Feeling and power of movement may be lost. The part appears stiff and white.

Do not rub the affected part. Do not apply direct heat in any form. Do not break any blisters

1 Shelter child from the weather. Give comfort and reassurance.

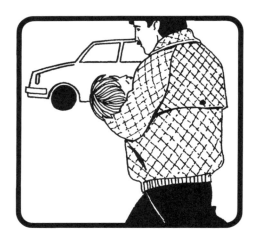

2 Give warm drinks if possible, but not alcohol.

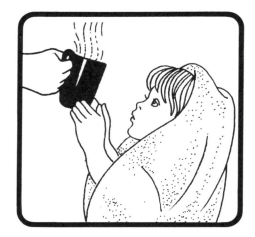

Frostbite

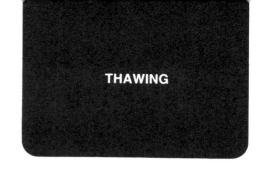

3 Remove constrictive clothing; eg gloves, rings, boots.

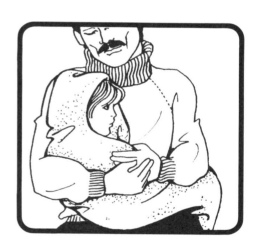

4 Thaw the affected part by warming gently with gloved hands, warm blankets or by placing the affected fingers under the armpit or wrapping in a sleeping bag. Continue until colour, sensation and warmth return to the affected parts. DO NOT massage.

5 Meanwhile, transport child to medical aid as soon as possible.

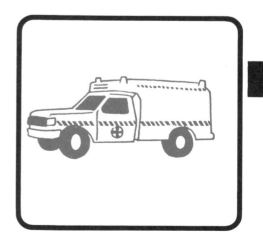

Head injuries

A moderate to severe blow on the head will usually cause a degree of concussion even if there is no damage to the underlying bone. **Symptoms** include: 'seeing stars'; temporary, partial or complete loss of consciousness; shallow breathing; nausea and vomiting; paleness; coldness and clamminess of the skin; later loss of memory.

Any case of unconsciousness must be referred to a doctor or hospital

1 Lay the child down and give warmth and comfort.

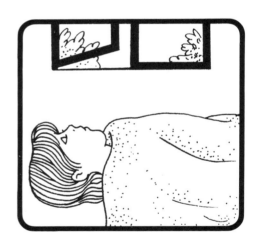

2 Do not give any drinks.

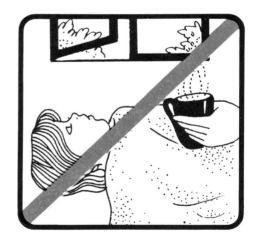

100

Head injuries

3 Apply a cold compress to the location of the blow or injury.

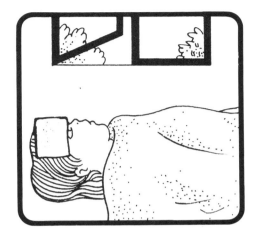

4 If unconsciousness develops, place the casualty in the lateral position (see page 17).

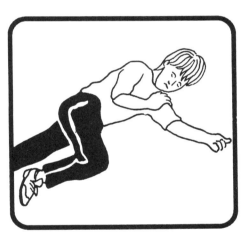

5 Observe for signs of more serious, deeper injury to the brain: deepening unconsciousness, persistent vomiting, double vision or persistent severe headache. Should any of these develop, remove child to hospital immediately by ambulance.

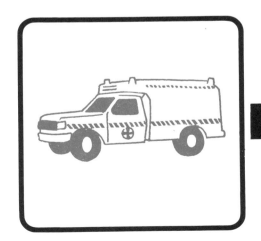

Head injuries

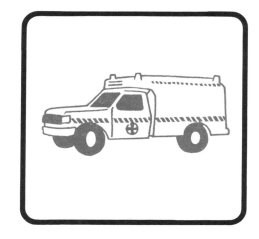

For anything but a small superficial cut or knock to the head, remove child to the nearest medical aid. Any tear or cut to the scalp or face tends to bleed heavily. Most are not serious although they look bad. Severe injury to the head can cause fracture of the underlying bones and in some cases injury to the brain.

1 Clean minor and superficial scalp and face wounds with soap and water.

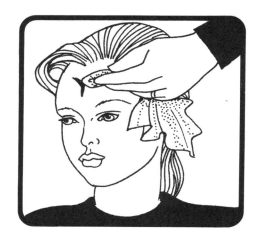

2 Compress the bleeding point with clean gauze or cloth until bleeding stops.

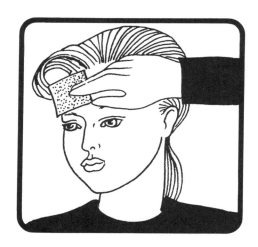

Do not give drinks after severe head injuries — sips only can be given

102

Head injuries

3 Cover, if necessary (and possible), with clean adhesive plaster.

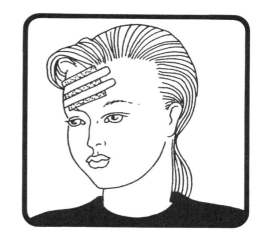

4 If the injury is more severe, lay the child down with head and shoulders propped up. Compress a large clean gauze or cloth lightly over the wound and attach with a bandage. Do not attempt to clean.

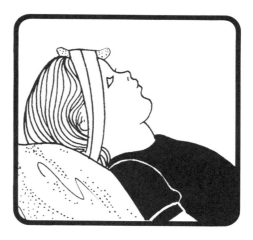

5 Watch the level of consciousness – see page 16. Check the pulse: if it stops apply heart compression – see page 12.
Watch for signs of shock and, if necessary give the treatment described on page 116.

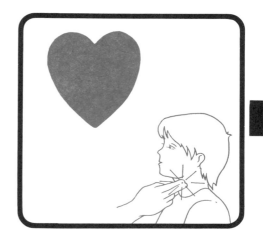

Impaled objects

Summon or transport to medical help immediately. Do not move a child off an impaling object unless his life is in imminent danger. If it is necessary, remove him as gently as possible. Do not attempt to remove the object unless it is obviously smooth and easy to do so. Otherwise, cut off any long projection 3-5cm from the skin surface. Try not to move the object.

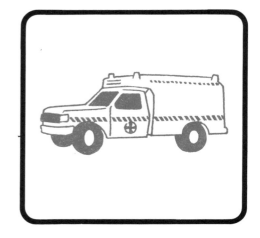

1 Cut clothing from around wound. If bleeding is severe see page 56.

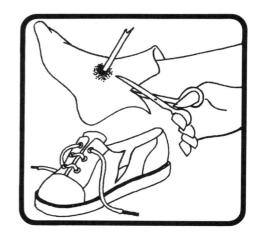

2 Place thick dry dressings around the wound and attach with bandaging.

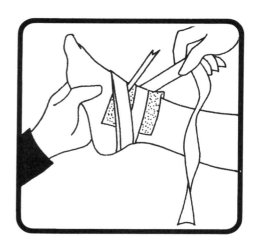

Watch the child for signs of shock. See page 116

104

Impaled objects

1 Do not attempt to remove a fish hook from a child's face. In other parts of the body, push the shank through the skin until the point appears.

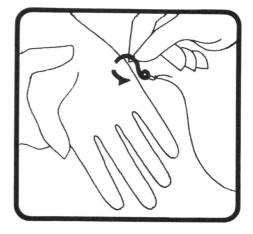

2 Cut off the barbed point with a wire-cutting tool. Retract the remaining shank from wound.

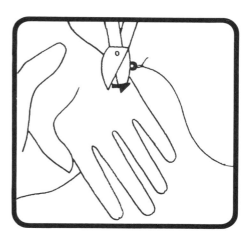

3 Clean the wound well with soap and water and cover with a clean dressing. Seek medical advice.

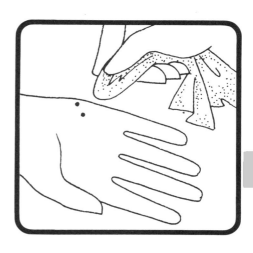

Mouth injuries

IMPORTANT

If bleeding has been severe or is not controllable, summon medical help. If the wounds are associated with other injuries see Head Injuries, page 100.

1 Clear the mouth of any broken teeth. If they are second teeth, wash with milk and replace into socket. If first teeth, control bleeding by pressure — do not replace teeth.

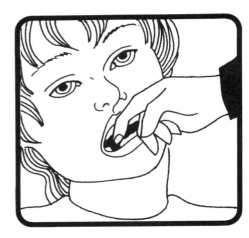

2 Sit the child down leaning slightly forward. Provide a bowl for the child to spit into.

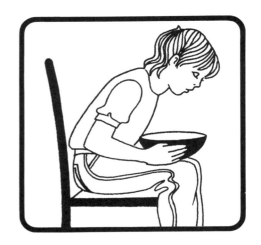

Mouth injuries

3 Apply direct pressure to tooth socket or wound by placing thick gauze or cotton wool pad firmly in position.

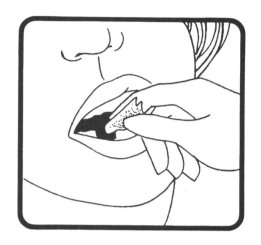

1 **TONGUE, CHEEK OR LIP**
Compress the bleeding part between the finger and thumb, using a clean handkerchief or gauze dressing until bleeding stops. Ask the child to bite down on the pad for 5 to 10 minutes, supporting his chin with his hand.

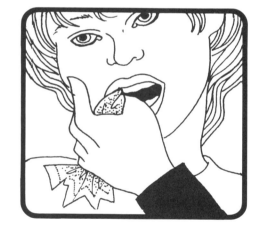

2 Do not wash out the mouth as this can disturb the clotting. Do not attempt to plug the socket.

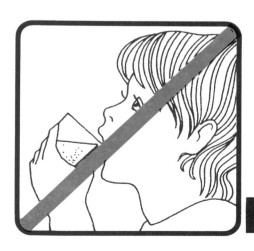

107

Poisoning

IMPORTANT

In all cases of poisoning, seek immediate medical help. Poisons may enter the body by being swallowed, inhaled, absorbed through the skin or injected under the skin. Swallowed poisons will have to be identified before the correct treatment can be given, but if in doubt, treat as corrosive poison.

1 Identify and keep safely the poison container. Save any vomit for later analysis. Do not induce vomiting.

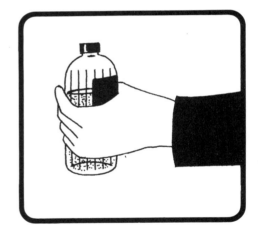

2 Telephone your local Poisons Information Centre, doctor, Hospital Emergency Department or Ambulance Service for advice.

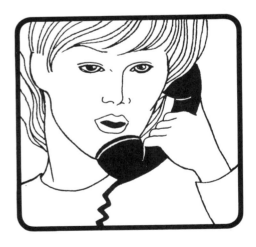

For a list of corrosive and non-corrosive poisons see page 121

Poisoning

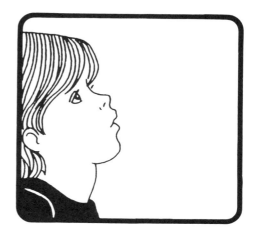

CORROSIVE POISONS

1 If child is conscious, give nil by mouth unless advised by medical aid. Loosen tight clothing and allow plenty of fresh air.

2 If unconscious, place in the lateral position (see page 17) and call immediate help.

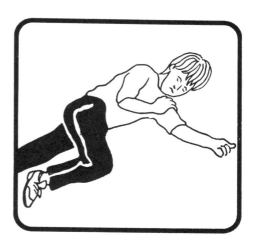

3 Treat for burns if necessary – see page 62.
Watch the breathing: if it stops give artificial ventilation — see page 10.
Check the pulse: if it stops apply heart compression – see page 12.

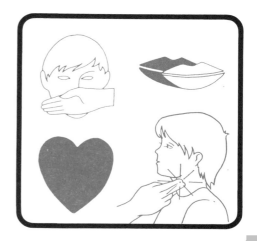

Poisoning

IMPORTANT

Summon immediate medical help. A list of non-corrosive poisons is given on page 121. If you suspect that a child has swallowed one of these, or any other poison, telephone your local Poisons Information Centre.

1

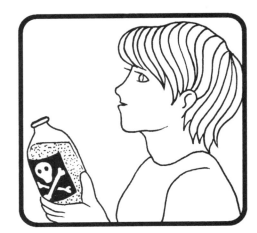

2

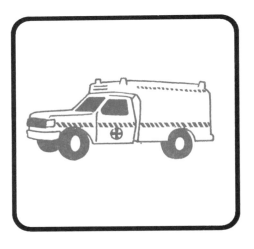

The procedure outlined on these pages also applies to swallowed poisonous plants – see page 122

110

Poisoning

3 If advised induce vomiting. Keep the child's head well down to avoid him inhaling any vomit.

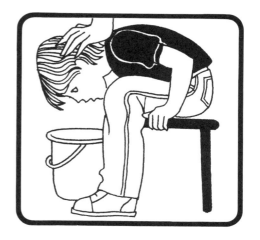

4 After vomiting save vomit for later analysis.

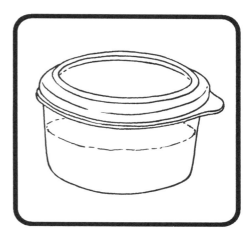

5 Watch the breathing: if it stops give artificial ventilation — see page 10.
Check the pulse: if it stops apply heart compression – see page 12.

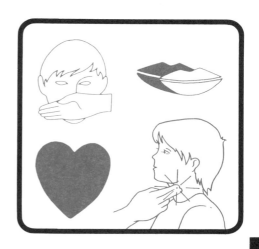

If there is any doubt about the poison which has been taken, act as described for corrosive poisons

Poisoning

This type of poisoning may be caused by gases, smoke from fire, solvents and certain paints.

If necessary, and possible, attach yourself to a life-line before entering a gas, or fume-filled space

1 **CAUTION:** Protect yourself — take a few deep breaths before entering a gas-filled room and take a deep breath and hold it when entering the room. A damp rag or handkerchief around your nose and mouth can help.

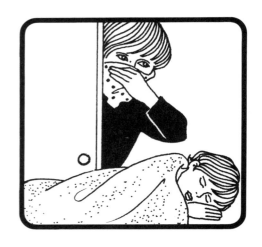

2 Immediately remove the child from the source of fumes and/or stop the source; eg stop car engine or turn the gas tap off.

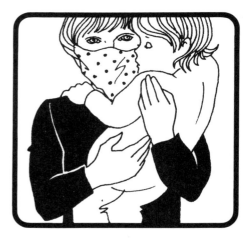

Poisoning

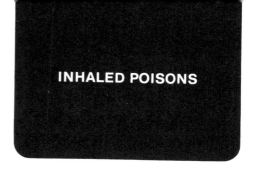

3 Loosen tight clothing and allow fresh air: open doors and windows.

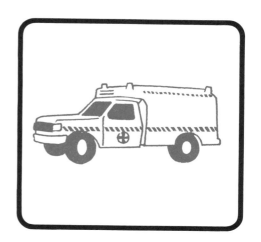

4 If child is affected or unconscious, remove child to hospital immediately. Complications may take some time to occur.

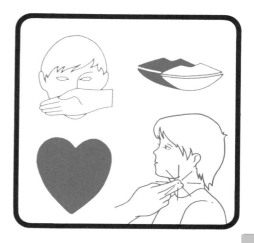

5 Watch the breathing: if it stops give artificial ventilation — see page 10.
Check the pulse: if it stops apply heart compression – see page 12.
Watch for signs of shock and if necessary give the treatment described on page 116.

Poisoning

Skin contact with certain plants can cause burning, itching, a rash, blisters, swelling, and sometimes headache and a fever.

For a list of poisonous plants see page 122

1 Remove the child from contact with the plant.

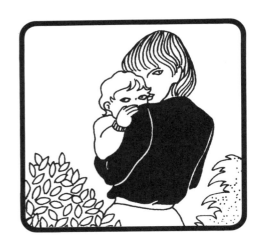

2 Wash the affected areas well with cold water and soap.

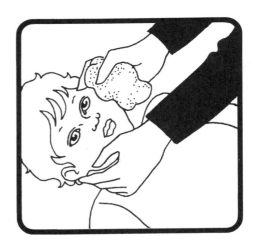

114

Poisoning

3 Apply calamine lotion or cologne. Antihistamine may be helpful if itching occurs.

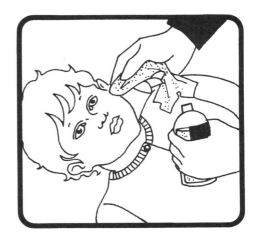

4 If the reaction is severe, seek medical advice.

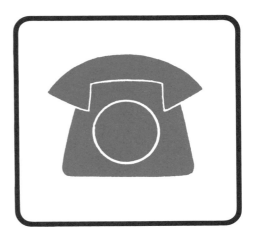

5 In known susceptible children — especially in those with severe allergy – transport to hospital immediately while watching out for shock and breathing difficulties. See page 16 or 116 if necessary.

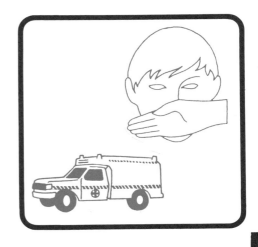

Shock

Symptoms: Usually the child becomes pale, the skin cold and clammy and there is usually sweating; sometimes giddiness, blurring of vision and vomiting. Drowsiness and unconsciousness may follow and the pulse, after becoming rapid, will be almost impossible to feel. Breathing may be rapid and shallow and may stop.

Do not overheat, as warmth draws blood into skin and away from vital organs. Do not give drinks — sips only

1 Lay the child down and deal with the immediate cause of shock. Move the child as little as possible.

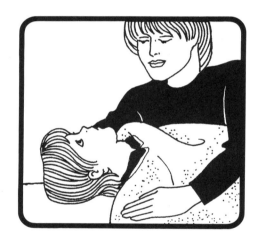

2 Loosen any tight clothing and allow plenty of fresh air.

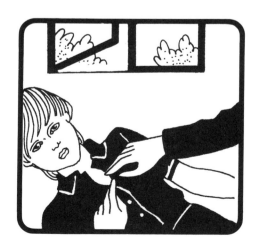

116

Shock

FOR RECOVERY

3 Keep the child's head flat and support the legs in an elevated position — this encourages blood flow to the brain.

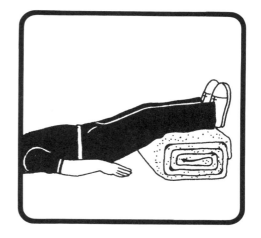

4 If vomiting seems likely or the child is unconscious, place in the lateral position — see page 17. Find a suitable pot into which the child can vomit.

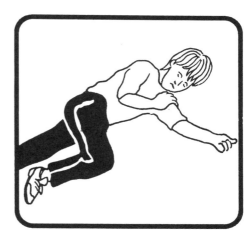

5 Summon medical aid as soon as possible.
Watch the breathing: if it stops give artificial ventilation —
see page 10.
Check the pulse: if it stops apply heart compression – see page 12.

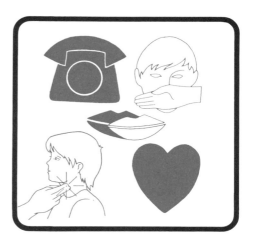

See Unconsciousness, page 16

SECTION 3

What you need to know

Children's medical history

Keeping a record of your children's medical history can save valuable time in an emergency. The chart on this page shows the kind of information which should be recorded. Keep the information up-to-date and provide copies for teachers, camp leaders or other adults who will be responsible for your children when they are away from home.

FAMILY NAME _____

FAMILY ADDRESS _____

	FIRST CHILD	SECOND CHILD
NAME		
DATE OF BIRTH		
NATURE OF BIRTH		
BREAST FEEDING UNTIL		
IMMUNISATIONS		
(See immunisation schedule)		
1st PDT + polio		
2nd PDT + polio		
3rd PDT + polio		
Measles		
Booster DT		
+ polio		
Booster tetanus		
VACCINATION		
BLOOD GROUP		
ALLERGIES		
MAJOR INJURIES		
HOSPITALISATION		
OPERATIONS		
MAJOR ILLNESSES		
PSYCHIATRIC CARE		
OTHER INFORMATION		

Emergency telephone numbers

A list of emergency telephone numbers is a vital part of your First Aid equipment. It is not sufficient just to keep the numbers of the police, fire and ambulance services – you never know when you may need one of the others listed here. Keep a copy of the list next to your telephone and show it to your babysitter whenever you go out.

YOUR DOCTOR _____

    Reserve Doctor _____

AMBULANCE _____

POLICE _____

FIRE STATION _____

DISTRICT HOSPITAL _____

CHILDREN'S HOSPITAL _____

DENTIST _____

CHEMIST: nearest all-night _____

FATHER'S WORK No. _____

MOTHER'S WORK No. _____

NEIGHBOURS and FRIENDS _____

    Name _____

    Address _____

    _____

    Telephone No. _____

    Name _____

    Address _____

    _____

    Telephone No. _____

TAXI _____

GAS _____

ELECTRICITY _____

WATER _____

OTHERS _____

For further advice and information on safety contact the following National Safety Councils in your capital city:

Queensland, NSCA (07) 252 8977
New South Wales, NSCA (02) 690 1555
Victoria, Victorian Safety Council Limited (03) 525 2255
South Australia, NSCA (08) 234 3034
Tasmania, NSCA (002) 23 2853
Western Australia, Industrial Foundation for Accident Prevention (09) 332 3511
Northern Territory, NSCA (089) 47 0404

Household poisons

Most households contain, in the form of quite ordinary substances, a surprising number of poisonous, or potentially poisonous, items. You cannot keep your house entirely free of such dangers, but you can ensure that they are kept under lock and key or out of your children's reach. Many poisons, especially petroleum products, must be kept well away from fire or naked flames.

The list below indicates a number of poisons which are found in very many households. For treatment of corrosive poisoning, see page 109; for treatment of non-corrosive poisoning, see page 110.

CORROSIVE
Battery acid
Benzine
Brush cleaner
Caustic soda
Charcoal lighter fuel
Corn remover
Dishwasher granules
Drain cleaner
Floor polish
Furniture polish
Gasoline
Grease remover
Gun cleaner
Kerosene
Lacquer thinner
Lye
Metal cleaner
Naphtha
Oven cleaner
Paint stripper
Paint thinner
Quicklime
Shoe polish
Toilet bowl cleaner
Typewriter cleaner
Wart remover
Washing soda
Wax wood polish
White spirit
Wood preservative
Zinc compounds

NON-CORROSIVE
Acetone
After shave lotion
Alcohol
Antifreeze
Arsenic
Bichloride of mercury
Bleach
Body conditioner
Boric acid
Camphor
Carbon tetrachloride
Chlordane
Cologne
Cosmetics
DDT
Deodorant
Detergent
Fabric softeners
Fingernail polish and remover
Fireworks
Fluoride
Hair dye
Hair permanent neutralizer
Hair sprays

Hydrogen peroxide
Indelible markers
Inks
Insecticides
Iodine
Liniment
Matches (more than 20 wooden matches or 2 match books)
Mercury salts
Mothballs, flakes or cakes
Nutmeg (if eaten whole)
Oil of Wintergreen
Paint (lead)
Perfume
Pesticides
Pine oil
Rat or mouse poison
Roach poisons
Strychnine
Suntan preparations
Turpentine
Weed killer
Wick deodorizer

For advice and information on poisons, phone the Poisons Information Centres in your state:
Queensland, Brisbane (07) 253 8233, country areas 008 177 333
New South Wales, Sydney (02) 692 6111, country areas 008 251 525
Victoria, Melbourne (03) 345 5678, country areas 008 133 890
South Australia, Adelaide (08) 204 6117, country areas 008 182 111
Tasmania, Hobart (002) 388 485, country areas 008 001 400
Western Australia, Perth (09) 381 1177, country areas 008 119 244
Northern Territory, phone NSW Poisons Information (02) 692 6111

Poisonous plants

The chief problem in warning of the dangers presented by poisonous plants centers around what is meant by poisonous. The list opposite, and the illustrated plants, can all be regarded as moderately to severely toxic — many of them can be fatal to children. Those with attractive fruits are a particular hazard to children. Children under the age of three should be kept away from obvious temptation; older children should be educated to recognise dangerous plants.

If you suspect that your child has consumed a poisonous plant, take a sample of the offending plant to the hospital with the child. Take an entire stem or branch together with flowers and fruits — if it has them.

FRUITS AND SEEDS

Abrus precatorius (Rosary pea)
Argemone (Mexican poppies)
Cestrum
Clivia (Kaffir lily)
Cotoneaster
Cycadales (Cycads, zamias)
Daphne
Delphinium
Duboisia (Corkwoods)
Hedera helix (English ivy)
Ilex aquifolium (Holly)
Jatropha
Laburnum
Lathyrus odoratus (Sweet pea)
Melia azerdarach (White cedar)
Papaver somniferum (Opium poppy)
Phytolacca americana (Pokeweed)
Pimelea flava (Yellow rice-flower)
Pimelea pauciflora (Scrub kurrajong)
Ricinus communis (Castor oil plant)
Solanum (Nightshades)
Thevetia peruviana (Yellow oleander)
Wikstroemia indica (Tie-bush)
Wisteria
Ximenia americana (Yellow plum)

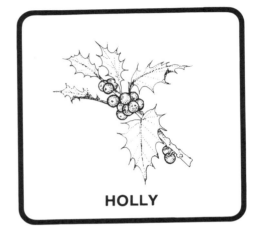

HOLLY

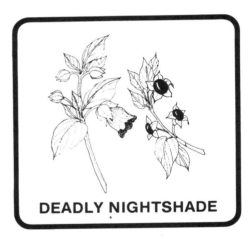

DEADLY NIGHTSHADE

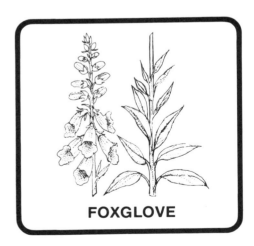

FOXGLOVE

Poisonous plants

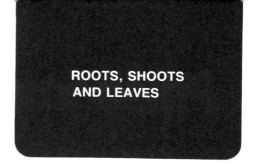

ROOTS

Aconitum (Monkshood)
Gloriosa superba (Glory lily)
Hyacinth (bulbs)
Manihot esculenta (Cassava)

FLOWERS

Gelsemium sempervirens (Yellow jasmine)
Kalmia latifolia (Mountain laurel)
Zantedeschia (Arum lily)

SHOOTS/FOLIAGE

Aesculus (Horse chestnut)
Buxus sempervirens (Boxwood)
Crinum (Spider lilies)
Dieffenbachia (Dumbcane)
Euphorbia (Spurges)
Hedera helix (English lily)
Laburnum
Philodendron
Rheum rhaponticum (Rhubarb – leaves only)

ALL PARTS POISONOUS

Atropa belladonna (Deadly nightshade)
Carissa spectabilis (Wintersweet)
Carissa acokanthera (Bushman's poison)
Conium maculatum (Hemlock)
Convallaria majalis (Lily-of-the-valley)
Datura (Thorn apples, false castor oil)
Digitalis (Foxglove)
Helleborus niger (Christmas rose)
Hyoscyamus niger (Henbane)
Ipomoea (Morning glory)
Ligustrum (Privets)
Lupinus (Lupins)
Narcissus (Daffodil, jonquil, narcissus)
Nerium oleander (Oleander)
Nicotiniana
Robinia
Taxus baccata (Yew)

POISONOUS ON CONTACT

Anacardium occidentale (Cashew)
Dendrocnide (Stinging tree)
Hoya Rhus
Sarcostemma astrale (Caustic vine)
Schinus (Pepper trees)
Synadenium granti (African milk bush)
Toxidendron (Poison ivy)

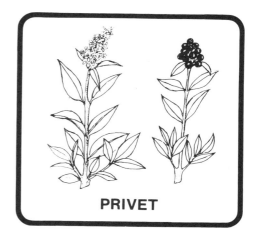

PRIVET

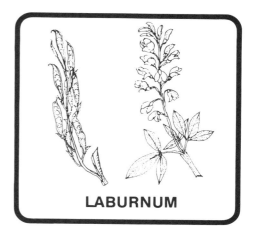

LABURNUM

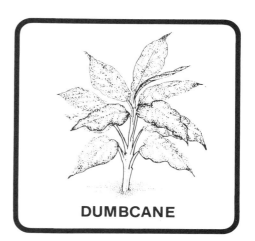

DUMBCANE

Poisonous snakes

Australia has the unenviable distinction of possessing around one hundred species of poisonous snakes, most of them belonging to a front-fanged group known as the *elapids.* The extent of their deadliness varies considerably and those with the most effective venom are not necessarily the most likely to bite. The thirty or so species of sea snake, for example, include many deadly types but swimmers are rarely bitten. Shown here are some of the commonest land snakes.

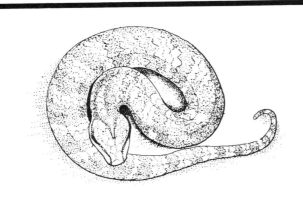

Death Adder — *Acanthopis antarcticus;* up to 90cm; found throughout Australia, except in central deserts and South Eastern NSW; body colour varies through shades of grey and brown with irregular cross-banding; nocturnal; often seems sluggish but strikes with great speed — usually only when touched.

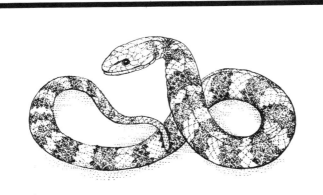

Tiger Snake — *Notechis scutatus;* up to 120cm; SE Australia and Tasmania; great variety of colours from pale grey to dark brown with yellowish cross-banding; not especially aggressive but extremely numerous and quite deadly.

124

Poisonous snakes

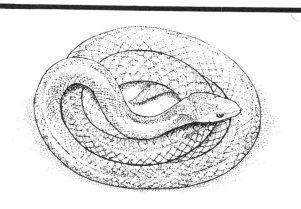

Taipan — *Oxyuranus scutellatus;* up to 400cm; confined to parts of Northern Australia, including Queensland; pale to dark brown, evenly coloured with yellowish area around head; extremely aggressive and given to unprovoked attacks.

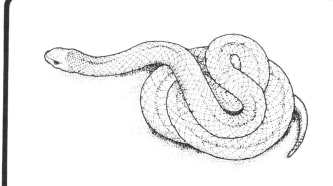

Brown Snake — *Pseudonaja textilis;* up to 160cm; found largely in NSW; variable colour, from light brown to a very dark shade, sometimes with cross-bands; a timid but very agile snake; because it inhabits the more densely populated parts of eastern Australia, it is responsible for a very high proportion of snakebite.

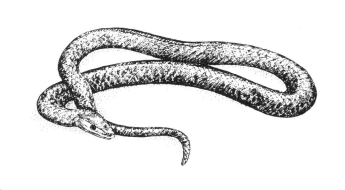

Red-bellied Black Snake — *Pseudechis porphyriacus;* up to 150cm; found along the entire East coast of Australia and in swamps and river flats throughout the South Eastern part of the continent; gleaming black body with red lower scales on the lateral surfaces; not very aggressive.

Index

Index